Solving the Puzzle of Chronic Fatigue Syndrome

Michael Rosenbaum, M.D. & Murray Susser, M.D.

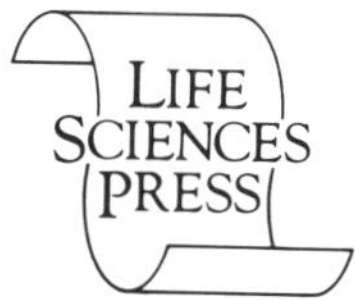

Life Sciences Press
Tacoma, WA

Disclaimer

While it may be your constitutional right to implement the methods described in this book, it is suggested that you not undertake any diet, nutritional regimen or program of exercise without the direct supervision of a licensed and fully qualified physician.

Life Sciences Press, P.O. Box 1174, Tacoma, WA 98401

Made in the United States of America

Third Printing, August 1996

Library of Congress Cataloging-in-Publication Data

Rosenbaum, Michael.
Solving the puzzle of chronic fatigue / Michael Rosenbaum, Murray Susser/
p. cm.
Includes index.

ISBN 0-943685-11-7 Soft Bound
ISBN 0-943685-15-X Hard Bound

1. Chronic fatigue syndrome.
I. Rosenbaum, Michael, 1942- . Susser, Murray, 1934- .

II. Title.
[DNLM: 1. Fatigue Syndrome, Chronic--etiology. 2. Fatigue Syndrome, Chronic--therapy. WC 500 R813s]
RB150.F37R67 1992
616'.047--dc20
DNLM/DLC
for Library of Congress 91-053018
CIP

DEDICATION

We dedicate this book to the memory of the late Dr. Norman Cousins. Norman was a colossus who bestrode the several worlds of medicine and literature simultaneously. Himself a victim of two severe diseases, he learned to deal with them using philosophies and technologies that we feel represent the spirit of this book. Dr. Cousins embraced standard medicine with one arm and ventured out into the frontiers of the alternatives with the other. He was constantly seeking. He would never stand pat with a weak hand. Dr. Cousins embodied the tough spirit of healing for which we constantly strive in our work and in this book. If we can follow the genius and loving example of Norman Cousins, we will succeed in assisting patients in rebuilding their lives.

Table of Contents

ACKNOWLEDGEMENTS

We wish to thank these special people for their vital contributions to the creation of this book. These friends and professionals contributed in much greater ways than we are able to mention in this brief tribute. These wonderful supporters are listed in un-alphabetical, random order.

Dr. Jack and Rose Herschorn, Barry Karr, Wayne and Hazel Birdzell, and Howard Colburn gave us invaluable help with our computer setups.

Phoebe Larmore gave us many ideas from her rich literary experience and much moral support from her richness of spirit.

Alan and Stacie Pando cheered us and steered us in the mysterious world of health literature.

Steve and Wanda Gilbert loaned us media smarts and sense of humor. We shall never repay them.

Dr. David Allen and Dr. Jeffery Anderson, our day to day associates, contributed daily knowledge and examples of exquisite patient care which broadened the scope of our experience in CFS. Dr. Mary Harper deserves a special note of gratitude and affection for contributing sanity throughout this arduous literary process and for clarifying the title of this book. Dr. Betty Kamen, a noted nutritionist and prolific writer, has been a continual source of inspiration and encouragement.

Dr. Hyla Cass constantly networked for us and brought us together with each other and many others. We gratefully acknowledge her enthusiastic support.

Dr. Dori Glover and Alan Galka provided cheerleading and clear perceptions when we needed them.

Dr. Jay Goldstein has been a special inspiration. His brilliant work in CFS and his dedication to solving this massive health problem gave us a gold standard by which to measure our work.

Dr. Mel Werbach is always an impeccable reference source and resource.

Pete Goodwin said it could be good financially if we sold a lot of books.

Vince Scully said we would have to pay taxes on it no matter what.

Dr. Eugene Landy and Alexandra Morgan gave us important ideas about the nature of stress and the psychology of fatigue.

Dr. Buddy Green and Dr. Cynthia Watson have been important contributors to our monthly doctor's study group. From them, we have gathered fresh information about Lyme disease and female disorders as well as numerous clinical pearls.

Betty Fredericks and Damien Simpson, at either end of the continent, are wise and knowing advisors.

A special note of appreciation goes to Stephen Clein for being the closest of friends and for always speaking the plain truth. We are O.K., just as we are.

We have formerly considered it somewhat corny to thank our patients who contributed to our experience in dealing with CFS. We have since changed our minds. We now know that the patients truly make this work possible. The confidence, which these people have bestowed on us, gave us the opportunity to practice our art and sharpen the skills that resulted in this book. We are humbly grateful to them for the trust and courage they have displayed. We thank them, each and every one.

Special Acknowledgement

We make special mention of Stephen Cherniske and Cindy Flinn Weeks. From the first, Steve made major contributions as consultant to the project. He worked diligently and effectively at many levels to bring this to life. Steve provided the early inspiration and know-how, without which this book would have never come to pass. Cindy is herself a recovered CFS sufferer. Cindy researched much of the scientific data which documents the information in the book. Her determination and attention to detail were of great benefit in the formative stages of this project. We are deeply grateful to Steve and Cindy

And to our publisher, Life Sciences Press, under the capable direction of Alexander Schauss and Laura Babin, we cordially tip our hats in grateful appreciation for their scientific knowledge, cooperation, prodding and kind understanding. We thank them both profoundly.

We owe the dazzling design of the bookcover to Sharon Wells, a recent graduate of the prestigious Art Center College of Design in Pasadena, CA, who graphically put the puzzle on paper.

Most Special Acknowledgement

We do most lovingly thank our ladies, Rodijah Peters and Phyllis Susser. It was no small task for them to suffer the deprivations required by this extended opus. With their love and support, their perception and intuition, they created the garden in which we could nurture and harvest our work. If the fruits of our labors do ultimately nourish people, it is because of this teamwork.

Thank you, thank you, and thank you kindly.

[P.S. Among the authors' offspring, there are 11 children, 2 sons-in-laws, 1 daughter-in-law, and 5 grandchildren. It behooves us, in the interest of family accord, to mention each one by first name only. Ivory, Crystal, Amber, Sharon, Julie, Todd, Joshua, Jenny, Justine, Mike, Janelle, Diane, Jeff, Bill, Andrew, Hayley, Caitlin, Melissa, and Spencer. We love you all and thank you for teaching us about fatigue in a most personal fashion.]

FOREWORD

The concept the Dr's Rosenbaum and Susser have of mixed infections and other factors altering the activity of the immune system and resulting in chronic fatigue is one which I believe will gain increasing acceptance in the 1990's. Patients do appear to have more immunologic disorders than previously and the suggestions about the reasons for this finding are quite provocative and worthy of consideration. The excellent results described for this diagnostic and therapeutic approach may gain adherents from physicians as well as patients who read this book. Some treatment-resistant conditions could be dealt with now, rather than waiting five or ten years until the proper experiments may or may not be done. The authors are to be congratulated on their inventiveness and their commitment to patient welfare in dealing with one of the most difficult medical problems of the late 20th century.

Jay Goldstein, M.D.

INTRODUCTION

Since 1985 we have been on a quest to help solve the puzzle of a mysterious epidemic called Chronic Fatigue Syndrome or CFS. We have felt an urgency to fit the puzzle pieces of this disease complex together because it devastates the health of vast numbers of people in the prime of their active lives for prolonged periods.

It is a most difficult puzzle to solve for many reasons. For one, its very existence has been denied by a large, skeptical sector of the medical profession as well as by social service agencies whose support is often desperately needed by CFS victims. It has been easy to scoff at the existence of CFS since it has no identifiable single cause. There is no simple test for it. Without a known cause or means of identification, there has been little chance of finding a "magic bullet" type of cure.

On the other hand, we have found a variety of causes and cures for patients who suffer from this multi-faceted disease. Our backgrounds are in preventive medicine. Our credo has been to shore up the body's own natural defenses against disease with proper diet, exercise, a healthy lifestyle, and the judicious use of nutritional supplements. We have been actively involved in treating CFS by this approach since it commanded public attention in 1985; actually, we have been treating CFS with this approach for about two decades—long before we had a name for it. For the past several years, we have collaborated in an ongoing effort to make sense out of this condition. Our spirited dialogue has reviewed many of the ongoing and nagging questions about Chronic Fatigue Syndrome:

Is CFS really just one disease caused by a single virus or by a family of viruses? Since it seemed to appear at the same time as AIDS, is a similar virus (retrovirus) involved in its transmission? Is this a mixed infection with many microbial players?

Is there an active infection after all?

Or, could CFS be primarily a disease caused by abnormal immune regulation with overproduction of vital immune chemicals called "cytokines" that make people feel sick?

Are there additional problems of hormonal imbalance, allergies, food and chemical sensitivity, and auto-immune reactions to complicate the symptom picture?

Is CFS just another name for depression or fibromyositis (inflamed muscles)?

Although unanswered questions abound, the good news is that many of the puzzle pieces of CFS can be identified and treated, providing relief to the patient. Although it is widely known that CFS is not life-threatening, many new patients are frustrated by the belief that "There is no cure for CFS." and are resigned to enduring years of exhaustion and disability with little help from the present medical approach.

We feel that Chronic Fatigue Syndrome is a complex disorder and must be looked at from a broad perspective of mixed infections, allergies, environmental illness, hormonal aberrations, stress, nutritional imbalances, and auto-immunity. CFS is not just depression! The puzzle is much larger than we originally anticipated. If some of these puzzle pieces can be properly identified and treated, the patient can obtain relief. Although, we cannot yet identify any single microorganism that may be the initial cause of the disease, we can identify and treat the bacteria, viruses, yeast and parasites that contribute to the total symptom picture. When we treat these organisms with specific antimicrobial measures, we often obtain good results. We can also intervene with nutritional therapy, hormone therapy, stress management, specific medications, and allergy treatments when appropriate. We can take measures to boost a sluggish immune response. We can offer hope to patients in despair.

IN THIS BOOK

In this book, we expand on the proposed major microbial players in the CFS story. We explore viruses, yeast, parasites, and bacteria in some depth. We discuss additional diagnostic possibilities including the concept of the Mixed Infection Syndrome (MIS) and enlarge on this idea in several chapters. It may be that much of what we now call CFS will ultimately be identified as a mixed infection complex.

We pay particular attention to the functions of the immune system. We feel that a simple working knowledge of how the immune system provides protection from disease and what we can do to enhance that protection can aid anyone with an infectious disease. We especially emphasize the individual nutrients, herbs and medications which help to correct specific immune imbalances.

We feel that the heart of the book and what really distinguishes it from most of the prior works on CFS, are the chapters on differential diagnosis (other potential causes) and treatment. Chapter 7 explains differential diagnosis and elaborates on the most likely other causes of CFS. If nothing else, this chapter can avoid the pitfall of misdiagnosing an obscure, but treatable condition that may be mistaken for CFS. Chapter 10 then gives a broad overview of treatment possibilities which far exceed what is now done by the ordinary medical approach.

The Appendix contains a unique feature which has drawn excited approval from those who have previewed the book: The flow chart series. We have developed graphic flow charts to simplify and organize the essence of the book. They can be used as a handy reference for both the professional and the lay reader. We intend that these flow charts, along with other aids which we have incorporated, will enhance the recovery of many CFS patients.

In the Appendix, we include a discussion of some of the salient points that emerged from the May, 1991 CFS conference (in Bel-Air, CA) inspired by Jay Goldstein, M.D.. Unfortunately, it was too late to incorporate this material into the main text of the book. The conference contained a lot of original and provocative information about CFS patients, including proof of abnormal blood perfusion in distinct areas of the brain, extremely high brain levels of an enzyme called RNAase which destroys the mechanism for memory storage and recall—and promising facts about Ampligen—a new drug currently undergoing research trials. Ampligen may soon prove to be the most potent single medication in the battle against CFS.

This conference included international leaders in the fight against CFS. Dr. Goldstein gathered outstanding workers such as Dr. Paul Cheney and Dr. Daniel Peterson, the physicians who originally described the disease at Incline Village, Nevada in 1984. Their presentations, as well as the brilliant and novel insights of Dr. Goldstein and the other presenters, provided increased clarity and the possibility of a long awaited solution to the CFS dilemma.

We are delighted to have Dr. Goldstein write the foreword. His own book, *Chronic Fatigue Syndrome - The Struggle for Health,* brilliantly describes CFS from a more traditional medical perspective. His theoretical genius has challenged us to probe much deeper into the brain-immune connection as it relates to CFS. Our approach should dovetail with the philosophy and science which Dr. Goldstein expounds. Even as we ponder our distinct differences of opinion, these serve to stimulate further our pursuit of ultimate truths about CFS.

Solving The Puzzle of Chronic Fatigue Syndrome answers pertinent questions while it poses others. The goal is to help CFS patients to improve their health and avoid some of the stigmata of this frustrating long term illness. We fervently hope that this book will spread some of the success that we have enjoyed with many of our CFS patients.

MICHAEL E. ROSENBAUM M.D. MURRAY R. SUSSER M.D.

CORTE MADERA & SANTA MONICA, CALIFORNIA October, 1991.

CHAPTER 1

THE PROBLEM

Feeling sick is an almost universal symptom in CFS...
25% of afflicted patients are bedridden, 40% can only work part time and only 35% can maintain a full time job.

A public health crisis has silently emerged during the past decade. It is called Chronic Fatigue Syndrome. This mysterious infectious illness has already drained the energy of an estimated three million Americans and ninety million people worldwide. It is an emerging epidemic which has been heralded as the "immune disease of the nineties!"

A prominent immunologist has estimated that there are five million exhausted Americans with undiagnosed Chronic Fatigue Syndrome. He further extrapolated that the incidence of Chronic Fatigue Syndrome is thirty times greater than multiple sclerosis, five times greater than Alzheimer's disease and a full ten times greater than than the number of people infected with the AIDS virus.

CFS has been overshadowed by the ominous spectre of AIDS. Both diseases appeared in the mid-nineteen seventies. Both are now recognized as acquired immunodeficiency disorders. AIDs is caused by an identified retrovirus which lives in our T-lymphocyte immune blood cells. It is a deadly disease. CFS does not kill but induces a lingering state of profound fatigue, malaise and weakness. The onset of this almost paralytic fatigue is often sudden. The average period of exhaustion is now estimated to last about two years!

CFS is a serious disease. Fifty percent of its victims are disabled and cannot work for varying periods of time. 25% of afflicted patients are bedridden, 40% can only work part time and only 35% can maintain a full time job.

The pattern of illness varies tremendously among individuals. Some are sick all the time. Others experience an ebb and flow with periods of remission alternating with periods of relapse.

The total length of illness varies as well. 1/3 of patients recover fully after only a few months; another third take a full two years to recover while the remaining third are still sick after two years.

It seems that women are more susceptible to CFS than are men. In America, 70% of CFS patients are educated and affluent Caucasian women in their childbearing years. This has prompted labels for CFS like the "yuppie flu" or the "Raggedy Ann Syndrome." It is unclear why women are more prone to the disorder. It is widely acknowledged that women are more health conscious than men and seek medical help more readily. There are other diseases which are known to predominate in women of childbearing age including Lupus, Rheumatoid Arthritis, Hashimoto Thyroiditis and Multiple Sclerosis. These diseases have a shared characteristic. They are all "auto immune" in nature, meaning that by some strange genetic quirk, the immune system attacks and destroys organs from its own body. Could CFS be an autoimmune disorder?

Most researchers point the guilty finger toward an as yet unidentified virus or family of viruses which lie dormant in the body and become "reactivated" at times of stress when the immune system falters. It is possible that CFS arises from a combination of infection and auto immunity. Multiple Sclerosis, as an example, is thought to be caused by a virus which infects brain cells and alters their surface in a way that "confuses" the immune system and provokes an autoimmune attack. It is intriguing that pictures of the brain performed by MRI (Magnetic Resonance Imaging) have revealed that CFS and MS patients seem to share a similar pattern of bright appearing lesions in the white matter of the brain.

Speculation and controversy still confound the CFS issue. Does the disease exist at all? Or, is it, as many stubborn physicians insist, another name for "depression" or "hysteria". If it does exist, is it caused by genetic damage to the immune system, by viruses or other infectious microorganisms or by an auto immune process? Or, by all three mechanisms combined? The jury is still deliberating.

FLU LIKE FEELING

Heather

Heather was the ideal young woman of the eighties. She was voted most likely to succeed in high school because of her take charge attitude and positive outlook on life. Add to this a warm smile and an endearing personality to make Heather a popular young lady.

In college, Heather exceled as an art student. She spent much of her free time painting and looked forward to a promising career in graphic design. As a Junior, she was awarded the University's art trophy. Heather was on top of the world. At least, for awhile.

At the end of her Junior year, during final exams week, Heather came down with a bad head cold and sore throat. She was feverish and achy. Somehow, she managed to pass her exams and looked forward to an exciting summer vacation. That summer, however, Heather needed much more sleep than usual and bed rest did not restore her energy. She began to feel exhausted. With the fatigue, came an overall flu like feeling with malaise, headache, body aches and muscle weakness. Aside from her lack of strength, Heather was tormented by a fear that she was "losing her mind" and would be forced to drop out of school. "I can't think anymore. I can't read more than a paragraph at a time. I lose my focus. Words seem to dance by on the page with no meaning. My memory is absolutely shot. I'm so frustrated. When is this illness going to end?"

Six months later, Heather still had to endure spells of malaise which persisted for weeks at a time. During these periods, every task seemed insurmountable. She would return home from school and would fall directly into bed and sleep through to the next morning. To make matters worse, her natural sparkle and charm seemed to disappear beneath a cloud of gloom.

Heather's doctors were stumped! Her blood count and general blood chemistry profile were normal. Special tests for arthritis and for various hormone levels were in the normal range. She was advised to see a psychotherapist. Three months of counselling did little to alleviate her distress. By the time she reached our office, Heather had all ready been ill for one year and was quite discouraged. "All I want to know is what I have. What is this disease?"

The condition that incapacitated Heather was virtually unknown until 1985 when two articles appeared in *The Annals of Internal Medicine* describing a mysterious flu like illness that had recently ravaged several population clusters in the United States. In one study, a symptom profile was developed which tabulated the percentage of patients affected by each symptom. Fatigue was the most common complaint, by far.

The breakdown was as follows:

Symptoms	**% of Patients Affected**
Fatigue	
easy fatiguability	95
fatigue alternating with periods of normalcy	70
can do usual work in spite of chronic fatigue	60
can work only part time	25
housebound	15
bedridden	15

Other Symptoms	**% of Patients Affected**
headache	80
low grade afternoon fever	78
swollen lymph glands	70
poor cencentration	70
sore throat	70
depression	70
allergies	65
muscle aches joint pains	50
anxiety attacks	50
mental confusion	50
sleep disturbance	50
abdominal problems	35
weight loss	20
skin rash	15

Fatigue is the hallmark symptom of CFS. In most surveys, a sense of profound fatigue occurs in almost 100% of respondents. And it is an easy fatigue. Minor exertion can cause major exhaustion! Light housecleaning or a short walk is all it takes to debilitate a CFS patient. It is not surprising that exercise actually makes a CFS patient feel much worse! People with CFS soon learn to cope with the disease by limiting their activity and by pacing themselves. A mid-day nap is often a necessity. Although bed rest is of benefit, it does not seem to rejuvenate. In common CFS parlance: "I sleep the day away and I'm still always tired!" CFS is much more than simple fatigue! A whole constellation of complaints occur which involve both mind and body. A sizable majority of patients have flu-like complaints including low grade afternoon fever, chills, sore throat, headache, body aches and joint pain.

Mental and emotional symptoms predominate. It is hard to think. The ability to concentrate is often impaired. Memory for recent events may be diminished. The brain seems to sputter as it would in a senile person. Imagine that someone is speaking to you. You may hear and understand the meaning of individual words but have to struggle to comprehend the message. Imagine further that you know what you want to say but the words come out wrong. The harder you try, the less sense you seem to make. Simply put, the brain is out of synch!

A majority of CFS patients exhibit elements of an organic brain syndrome. A test of memory function was conducted at The University of California on CFS patients. Depressed patients and healthy volunteers served as controls. The results, summarized in *Medical World News* (April 9, 1990) showed that CFS patients lagged behind controls and depressed patients. They could not record memories as efficiently as the others and were 21 times slower at mental scanning. Neuropsychology tests of CFS patients often reveal deficits in the ability to think and communicate. As previously noted, brain lesions often appear on MRI scans. These resemble the scattered bright appearing lesions in the white matter of the brain observed in Multiple Sclerosis. The scattered pattern of lesions may account for the wide variety of mental aberrations that occur in the Chronic Fatigue Syndrome. They may also account for the astounding 40 to 50% of CFS patients who have a balance disorder and who find it difficult to stand straight with their eyes closed or feel as if they are veering to the right or left when walking.

THE CONTROVERSY

The symptom picture in CFS is so extensive and diverse that it makes the disease difficult to diagnose. The very existence of CFS is still shrouded in controversy. Critics contend that CFS is a non-disease. In their view, the term CFS is a misnomer for several well known psychiatric disorders including hysteria, anxiety and depression. After all, mental illness is often accompanied by fatigue, loss of appetite, a sleep disturbance and brain fog. On the other hand, depression is not ordinarily characterized by flu-like symptoms including fever, chills, swollen glands or brain lesions all of which seem to set the CFS syndrome apart as a distinct clinical entity.

Detractors also point out that CFS is not a new disease. They claim that it is an old disease in new clothing and was first described in the medical literature one hundred years ago with the label "neurasthenia," a type of neurosis with accompanying depression. Over the years a number of other titles and causes have been assigned to this condition (which has, in their view, created an ongoing state of confusion), including: "hypoglycemia," "food allergy" and "Candida Hypersensitivity Syndrome." Proponents of a viral etiology named the disease "post viral fatigue syndrome." This label stuck until the mid-nineteen eighties when the first published reports linked CFS to the Epstein Barr Virus (EBV), known to be the cause of mononucleosis. That ushered in several new labels: "Chronic Mononucleosis Syndrome," "EBV," Chronic Fatigue Immune Dysfunction Syndrome (CFIDS), and "Chronic EBV"(CEBV). In Europe, a similar disease epidemic was named "Benign Myalgic Encephalomyelitis or BME." Another group called it "Icelandic Disease."

In an attempt to avoid confusion, the Center for Disease Control (CDC) in Atlanta created a working case definition of CFS in 1988. The major criteria include:

"New onset of a debilitating fatigue which must persist in a steady or relapsing course for at least six months and curtail average daily activity more than fifty percent."

"The exclusion of other medical conditions that produce similar complaints to CFS, including auto immune diseases such as lupus and rheumatoid arthritis; other chronic infections of a viral or non-viral nature (caused by bacteria, yeast or parasites) AIDs related disease, psychiatric disorders, neuromuscular and hormonal disorders."

"Minor criteria including low grade fever or chills, sore throat, swollen glands, muscle aches or weakness, joint aches, sleep disturbance, mental confusion, headache and emotional imbalance."

Malaise is not included in the criteria but definitely should be. Feeling sick is an almost universal symptom in CFS.

CDC CRITERIA UNDER ATTACK

The CDC case definition was a valiant attempt to set diagnostic guidelines for this disease. The criteria came under stern attack by researchers who met at an international conference on CFS in April, 1990 in Los Angeles.

What has been most criticized is the exclusion clause which makes it mandatory to consider first and exclude a large number of other possible causes before making a diagnosis of CFS. It is time consuming and costly to test every patient with CFS complaints for a long list of maladies. "The long list of exclusions makes it almost impossible to meet the criteria." said Dr. Don Goldenberg, Professor of Medicine at Tufts University in Boston. He further stated that "basically no one would have Chronic Fatigue Syndrome by the CDC criteria."

IMMUNE DYSREGULATION

One possible flaw in the CDC definition is that it considers only a single infectious agent as the cause for CFS, as if all other diseases are mutually exclusive. Actually, CFS can coexist with a broad spectrum of other diseases. This is especially true for conditions in which the immune response is weak, as in AIDS and in malignancies. There is also a popular theory that a dysregulated immune system is the underlying cause of CFS. The dysregulation could be caused by a virus or perhaps by toxic environmental chemicals which contaminate the immune system and scramble its messages.

That leads us into a century old controversy about the nature of communicable disease: microbe vs. host resistance. Does the infectious agent itself cause us to feel sick or do we succumb to illness because our immune system has been damaged? In the late nineteenth century, Pasteur advocated the single agent theory of infection which incriminated specific microscopic villains. Treatment approaches were therefore aimed at the identification and eradication of these microorganisms. Bechamps, on the other hand, claimed infection stemmed from weakened host resistence: "the soil, not the seed," was his position. With the recent resurgence of preventative medicine, there is a renewed appreciation of the vital role played by host resistance. The immune system is highly complex and dynamic. Malnutrition, stress and environmental pollution can damage the immune sensitive components and make us susceptible to infection.

As a result of this new way of thinking, considerable efforts are being directed toward biological ways of modulating the immune response. Immunomodulation with drugs and nutrients which are called biological response modifiers has become a mainstay of our treatment approach. (See Chapter 10 for details about the treatment program).

The single agent theory of infection has monopolized medical thinking during most of the twentieth century. As physicians, we have been trained to confront an infection by first obtaining a culture specimen from the zone of infection. The specimen is then incubated in a special culture medium in order to grow it out and identify it. An appropriate antibiotic may then be prescribed to destroy it.

ONE CAUSE
ONE SOLUTION
SIMPLE!

Unfortunately, there is no simple cure for the Chronic Fatigue Syndrome. To date, no single causative agent has been identified. The concensus is that a virus or group of viruses is involved. Most speculation has centered on the Herpes family of viruses which include the Epstein-Barr Virus (EBV), Cytomegalovirus (CMV), Herpes Simplex Viruses (oral and genital) and the Herpes Virus type-6.

The medical articles that opened the CFS Pandora's box in 1985 pointed the finger at EBV as being the culprit since the disease was thought of as being a chronic mononucleosis syndrome. There had been ongoing speculation through the years that "Mono" could recur, sometimes much later in life.

How can a virus survive in our body in a latent state for so many years? After all, bacteria have abbreviated lifespans and can be easily annihilated with the right choice of antibiotic. On the other hand, viruses are difficult to eradicate. First of all, viruses are not really alive. A virus is a packet of genetic material protected by a protein and lipid envelope. When a virus penetrates into a human cell, the surrounding envelope is extruded, releasing the viral genes which then incorporate into human chromosomes. Hovering within the nucleus of the human cell, viral genes are shielded from an immune attack. Some viruses can establish lifelong residence inside the human host. This is especially true of the Herpes viruses. Herpes simplex can lie dormant inside nerve cell ganglia for prolonged periods in a latent state and reemerge in a "reactivated" state when host resistance drops. EBV houses itself primarily in white blood cells called "B Lymphocytes," cells which are capable of manufacturing antibodies. EBV infection is known to upregulate the immune response by increasing the number of active B cells. EBV can also emerge and reinfect much later in life.

What prods these viruses out of hibernation? Do they suddenly become more virulent? Or, does a faulty immune system fail to contain them? There is growing respect for the belief that an immune breakdown occurs in the early stages of CFS. (The details of this breakdown will be elaborated in chapter 8.) The cause of the immune dysregulation is unknown. It has been suggested that a retrovirus, in the same general family as the AIDS virus, comes along and disrupts the rhythm of the immune response. Herpes viruses and other microbes are then free to flourish in what constitutes a mixed infection.

RUNNING ON EMPTY

CFS is not limited to the fairer sex. Although the disease seems to predominate among women, the incidence among the sexes or among age groups has been impossible to establish due to a lack of accurate diagnostic criteria. CFS definitely does occur in men of all ages and its effects upon social relationships and family finances are devastating for both sexes.

Robert G. is a good example. He was 51 years old when he first came to us for help in 1988. Robert had been a very successful businessman in New York City for fifteen years. With true "Type A" drive and ambition, he had worked his way to the top echelon of a prosperous textile manufacturing plant.

> *"I was under tremendous stress during those years. You might say that I was driven. For the first ten years, I worked ten to twelve hours a day and six hours a day on weekends. I never took a day off! But, I was doing so well, I didn't care. My energy was great and my mind was sharp."*
>
> *Five years ago, Robert decided to move to California to expand his business. Things progressed well until 1987 when his 61 year old brother, who was still living in New York City, suffered a heart attack. For the next three months, Robert lived a bi-coastal existence. He ricocheted between New York and California every week.*
>
> *"That is when I hit the proverbial brick wall. I got really tired. It felt like no matter how much sleep I got, it was never enough. My arms and legs felt sore and heavy all the time. It was like nothing I had ever experienced. There were times that just to drag my body out of bed to visit the bathroom took a superhuman effort. Every part of me ached. I knew that I was sick because this was much more than feeling run down. For a time, my nose ran, I had a sore throat and the sweats. What was so frightening is that my doctor didn't know what I had. Antibiotics were worthless. All the usual blood and culture tests came out normal. But, I was getting worse!*
>
> *Then my mind began to go. It happened a little bit at a time. At first, I had difficulty focusing on written material. I found myself re-reading the same paragraph in the morning sports section so often that I gave up on reading. I still felt that I had a flu that was hanging on and that I would improve shortly with rest. So, I tried to cut down my activities, although I still spent my days consulting with clients on the phone in bed. I had no idea how sick I really was until I reached a point when I could no longer conduct any business at all. There were days that I*

couldn't even add two and two. I could not recall routine facts like names of my personal friends. That got to be very embarrassing!

My handwriting also got very strange. My letters became smaller and I found myself struggling to spell simple words. At times, I would reverse letters in words or leave key words out of sentences. Although I could think of a word in my mind, somehow I couldn't write the word on paper. It was wierd!"

Two years later, Robert is still out of work. He was fortunate to own a piece of his old business. Otherwise, he would have been ruined financially. His social life had come to a standstill. It was too much effort to try to carry on a conversation without betraying his loss of brainpower. What made it so much harder was the fact that nobody seemed to understand. His doctor and even his best friends and family had doubts about his sincerity. A lot of people thought that he was faking it to get sympathy or get out of work.

The saga of Robert G. is common among CFS patients. He became frail abruptly and had not fully recovered in three years. He complained about a wide range of flu-like symptoms including profound fatigue, a nagging sense of malaise with muscle weakness and mental confusion. He could no longer work or maintain an active social life. And he was frightened because no one seemed to understand what he had or how long he would have it.

By the time he came to our office Robert had already been disabled for two years. The only medical treatment he had received was an anti-depressant prescribed by his family doctor. This medication did help to lift his mood but did nothing for his flu-like complaints. A comprehensive battery of laboratory tests revealed high antibody titers to the "early antigen" of the Epstein Barr virus (EBV), to the Cytomegalovirus (CMV), and to the Herpes virus type-6. Since these viruses have been the leading suspects for causing CFS, it was not surprising to see all three of them elevated in this patient.

Robert's immune blood tests were also abnormal in a way that typifies CFS patients. His Natural Killer Cells (NK) were sparse and he was lacking in the major subclass of IgG antibody, IgG-1, a vital defense against viral infection.

With a low immune reserve, Robert had become susceptible to a variety of other infections. A stool purge test for parasites revealed some roundworms, a microscopic organism called "Blastocystis" (commonly observed in CFS patients), and a lot of yeast cells. He figured that might explain his recurrent abdominal problems with bloating, constipation alternating with diarrhea and rectal itching. In addition, he became more prone to routine flus which incapacitated him far longer than usual. Old herpes eruptions began to resurface painfully around his lips and tongue.

Robert had a MIXED INFECTION.

It is our contention that many CFS patients are suffering from a Mixed Infection Syndrome (MIS) involving many microbial players which include viruses, yeast, parasites and bacteria. The mechanism for how this disease develops is unclear. According to our current analysis, the following schema might apply:

1. A virus, possibly a retrovirus, invades white blood cells and disorders the immune response. There may exist a genetic susceptibility to this 'initiator' virus. Environmental factors which can further dysregulate the immune response can be factored into this category and include malnutrition, exposure to pollutants in air, water and food and the use of immuno-supressive drugs.

2. Latent viruses, often of the Herpes family, can become reactivated and precipitate the Chronic Fatigue Syndrome.

3. A variety of other infections can ensue which further stress the immune response and add more weight to an already heavy symptom load. This is the *Mixed Infection Syndrome*.

CHAPTER 2

MIXED INFECTION SYNDROME and CFS

"Imbalance is the cause of all disease." *Anonymous*

Mixed Infection Syndrome (MIS) — definition: Debility caused by multiple, simultaneous and synergistic infections.

We must remember that every infectious disease that we now readily recognize, was once an obscure entity. Debility of obscure infectious origin is common, and those who suffer it are not only sick, but often abused by the health care system. If, as we have observed, CFS patients often suffer from one or more obscure infections, it is unconscionable to label them hypochondriac, malingerer, hysteric, or with the other pejorative misdiagnoses that have sprung up to meet the present immaturity of the standard medical approach to this problem.

We must attend to sick people who get little relief from the present conventional approach. The problem is that the conventional orthodox approach to disease is to identify a single cause. It is not a law of nature that every disease syndrome must have a single cause. Syndromes may have multiple causes. We appreciate that the conservative medical community has made major contributions to the standardization of health care. This standardization is a two edged sword. It gives the system stability, but by its very nature, it must restrict progress. While standard medicine delineates the cause and cure of newly recognized diseases, it often stifles imaginative therapy. Most observers recognize that standard medicine often gets its most crea-tive advances from non-standard ideas. Some medical theorists claim that is, in fact, the only way to have creative advances.

In our experience, CFS patients reveal a high degree of MIS. The infections which we most commonly find are yeast and parasites.

YEAST INFECTION

The presence of yeast in CFS infection is, as we have said, controversial because most of the medical community still does not recognize this insidious and prevalent infection. This infection has been brilliantly described by many researchers including Orion Truss, M.D. in his book *The Missing Diagnosis*, William Crook M.D. in *The Yeast Connection* and John Trowbridge M.D. in *The Yeast Syndrome*. Marjorie Crandall, Ph.D. has done exquisite work showing the connection between Candida hypersensitivity and CFS. Candida infection is a major part of the Mixed Infection Syndrome. When treated properly, its victims have gotten wondrous relief from malaise and chronic fatigue (see Chapter 4).

PARASITES

Parasites play a surprisingly large role in the CFS problem. Intestinal parasites are much more prevalent than most doctors have heretofore suspected. We believe that parasites are present in a large percentage of patients who complain of fatigue.(see Chapter 5.) For now, we should note that these common organisms are usually overlooked and ignored by the standard medical approach to CFS. When we discover and treat these parasite infestations, the chronic fatigue and attendant symptoms often improve or even disappear.

YEAST AND PARASITES

The concurrent presence of yeast and parasites is a form of MIS. Note that yeast and parasites are often treatable with standard medical drugs. We repeat: Treating these infections may give improvement or sometimes total relief to CFS patients.

DEPRESSION

Not surprisingly, many CFS patients get relief from their mental depression with successful treatment for MIS. It is not a big surprise to observe emotional depression in a CFS patient. Has anyone ever had an illness that was not at least a little depressing. It is depressing to be sick. When you are sick, you generally feel sick (malaise), and you have fatigue. Fatigue, malaise, depression, and cloudy thinking are nearly universal symptoms of systemic infection. Many CFS patients have been diagnosed as being "clinically" or "medically" depressed. We have treated many of these people for their obscure or ignored infections and their clinical depressions melted away as if by magic.

Example:

L.S. was a 29 year old professional writer. She was charming, attractive, inquisitive, and rather charismatic. Despite these assets, she was not healthy. On a scale of one to ten, she rated her energy at about two. She had enjoyed good health until age 27 when her health deteriorated abruptly. She suffered episodes of mental confusion, malaise, depression, panic attacks, severe intestinal pain, gas and nausea. She had sore throats, joint pain, rectal itching, and an almost constant feeling of Pre-Menstrual Syndrome (PMS). She had gradually become intolerant of many foods, especially fruits, dairy products, and wheat—all of which would exacerbate many of her symptoms.

Her story could fill an entire book by itself. In outline, she suffered from Candida overgrowth and had high blood antibody levels to Candida. She was found to have two kinds of intestinal parasites, namely *Giardia lamblia* and *Entameba histolytica*. The same stool tests revealed the presence of excessive Candida which tended to affirm the high antibody levels in her blood. She had also developed several dental abscesses which had gone unnoticed. Her antibody levels against Epstein-Barr virus (EBV) were significantly elevated. Other significant laboratory abnormalities included an elevated Erythrocyte Sedimentation Rate (ESR or "Sed Rate,"), which indicates non-specific inflammation, and a low Glycohemoglobin which indicates low blood sugar.

L.S. had been to many physicians, some of whom had helped somewhat; some, she felt, had worsened the problem with anti-depressent drugs and several of the other medical therapies which were being used at that time. By using nutritional therapies, she had reduced some of the symptoms, but not eliminated any of them. We did further studies. We discovered the intestinal parasites and defined the other problems already mentioned. We treated her with a veritable armada of therapies. She, of course, had diet therapy and vitamin and mineral supplements. She took full courses of four antiparasitic drugs, namely metronidizole, iodoquinal, Atabrine®, and Furoxone®. She completed courses of Nystatin to control the intestinal yeast. Her dental abcesses were drained and her dental problems were treated appropriately. She had to use antibiotics to assist the dental surgery. Space does not permit us to enumerate all the details of this long and painful story.

Suffice it to say that she gradually achieved good health. After two months of treatment, her energy had risen to about six out of ten (from her original two). Over a two year period, most of her medical problems came under control. Her food sensitivities and all of her other symptoms became almost insignificant. They became minor nuisances which barely bothered her—mere reminders of her former nightmarish ill health. It was not a simple and obvious cause and effect such as we like to see in medicine.

But watching her gradual return to the land of the living was a wonderful validation of much of the work that we do. The problems which she suffered are daily events in our practice. L.S. is somewhat unusual in that she had stubborn cases of yeast, parasites, bacteria and virus. Her illness was a fairly drastic example of the Mixed Infection Syndrome.

What lessons can we learn from this case? First, let us assume that the obvious is true. Let us say that this patient truly suffered from all of the conditions which the medical work-up revealed. Let us also say that the persistent MIS contributed to the CFS, the depression, and most of the other symptoms. It follows then, that the treatment of the infections worked and ultimately resolved this patient's depression and fatigue. In the context of CFS, this case could teach us many lessons:

1. CFS is not a simple disorder. We use this case to show how complex it can be.
2. Standard doctors who limit themselves to drug-of-choice therapy, may miss the diagnosis of infection.
3. We should do everything within reason to find hidden infection or some other hidden cause, when the patient has CFS.
4. One case report is only an anecdote. It has no scientific validity. It does not prove a point. *But it may be true!*

   We can draw conclusions, realizing the lack of science, on several thousand cases. We can use that information to treat other patients. It becomes part of our experience and our learning. Our future patients with CFS (with or without evidence of infection) should get a stool test and other tests to clarify the full extent of the mixed infection.
5. We should also realize that even with strong evidence as in this case, MIS may not have been involved in this patient's CFS.
6. Ideally, we would like to be able to study such cases with double-blind studies and other statistical methods. This

kind of research is expensive. A private practitioner cannot afford to do this alone. It is the province of a government or university or charitable foundation.

7. If we accept the cause of her fatigue as MIS, one could argue that this case was not an example of CFS; it was a case of amebiasis, giardiasis, yeast, bacterial abscess, EBV, and allergy. Therefore, we have six true medical diseases which by definition cannot be called CFS. Until a specific cause of CFS is found, we could argue endlessly whether this is CFS. Pigeon-holing is nice, but it should not get in the way of curing the patient.
8. Hidden infections can cause "clinical depression."
9. A mysterious shift in a patient's personality is not always due to some nebulous psychological cause.
10. As complex as this case is, some doctors might obscure its meaning by glibly writing it off as psychosomatic. We must avoid that trap.

There are certainly many possible interpretations of this case. In our experience, there are many similar cases which in our mind makes it likely that MIS caused the depression, and the treatment cured both problems. If that be the truth, think how many people with parasites and similar problems are suffering from misdiagnosed "clinical depression!" It is staggering.

We are going to make an important assumption. We are going to assume that in finding and treating one infection, we may often be treating other infections as well. The reason for this assumption is based on our experience that if we do not support the patient's immune response when we treat a single infection, the patient may not improve. On such occasions, further study may detect another infection; treating that infection turns the corner, and recovery soon follows. A slight perplexity occurs when we treat one infection, and the patient gets better. Did that patient only have one infection, or were there other infections which the body was able to master after the major infection was eliminated? This is only an academic point of interest. When the patient gets better, there is little care whether there was one or one hundred infections originally. We predict that when diagnostic technology improves, we will find many mixed infections which plague CFS patients to greater or lesser degrees.

Deficiency and Toxicity, the twin highwaymen of illness, lead to infections with resident and invasive viral, fungal, bacterial, and parasitic infections—often set against a background of allergy. Additionally, there is a "cumulative immune stress," often worsened by the emotional overlay of the infectious process. There is also the added burden of everyday stress which many CFS people cannot manage. There are synergistic relationships among all these causative entities.

Think of it this way. If you cut your skin, all the resident bacteria that are normally harmless bystanders suddenly become potential invaders. The bacteria begin to feed on you (ghastly concept); they invade your tissues, and you are infected. If some similar process should happen in your gut or your throat or anywhere in the body, how would you know? If there is a low grade yeast or parasite infestation of your intestines, and the infection becomes chronic, it may be impossible to test with our present clinical technology. It will definitely be impossible to locate, if the doctor does not have a clue that a parasite or yeast could be the cause. Discovery begins with suspicion. The doctor must have an index of suspicion or the disease will not be discovered.

Mixed infections often coexist with other diseases like rheumatoid arthritis and cancer. The terminal event of cancer is often a fulminent mixed infection; that is well known. What is not recognized is that early in a malignancy, the patient can have a low grade MIS that is undiagnosed. Once the patient has cancer, that cancer gets blamed for any symptoms that may occur. If the cancer patient has MIS as well as CFS, who would look for it? On the other hand, there are many cancer patients who feel fine, even into fairly advanced stages of the disease. It may be that they have not developed an MIS.

MIS is a big picture disease. Clearly, it is important to view the whole picture and treat all the underlying infections. We know that the *one drug to kill one germ* treatment often results in an overall worsening of CFS. Microorganisms not only coexist, they may encourage each other to grow. Candidiasis, for example, may cause staph infections. In a recent study it was discovered that individuals with a history of recurrent bacterial infection were found to have increased susceptibility to severe EBV disease.

Did immune weakness cause the bacterial infections, or did the treatment of the infections disrupt the immune system? Is it a vicious cycle? While researchers ponder the synergy of bacterial and viral infection, we suspect that immune dysregulation is a contributing factor. In addition, we also consider an indirect connection: EBV may proliferate to pathologic levels as a result of repeated bacterial infection and antibiotic therapy—and sometimes just one such course can initiate the problem. EBV proliferation, therefore, may be a barometer of immune weakness. The picture is large, involved and still unclear. It leaves us with questions.

It is fair to say that there are two questions which we need to answer about every disease:

1. What is it?
2. How do we cure it?

Since we cannot yet answer #1 for CFS, we may be in the strange position of truly putting the cart before the horse. We can sometimes answer #2. We often cure it. We also know that "often" is far from "always." Until we can always cure a disease, we must continue to seek the answer to #1. In later chapters, we will weave our plan for continuing to seek the cause, while we do our best with empirical treatment.

In the following chapters, we will address the individual organisms which participate in MIS and therefore much of CFS. Following that, we will examine the causes and treatments of immune system dysregulation, thereby tying it all together in a productive approach to CFS. It is our contention that by this global concept of the disease, we can get good therapeutic responses from patients. We do not propose to wait for the final explanation of the precise nature of CFS. Either it is caused by a single agent or it is not. Whatever the case, our patients get better at a faster rate than do the patients using the standard medical model. That to us is the central issue.

CHAPTER 3

VIRUSES and RETROVIRUSES

We believe that the job of medical researchers is to look beyond the narrow single-cause model of disease... viruses often act in concert with other pathogens in causing disease.

This book is about the multitudes of people worldwide who seem to hit a brick wall often in the third to fifth decades of life. Their story of recurrent flu-like complaints including profound fatigue, malaise, fever and body aches has convinced many that a virus is the major cause of CFS. So far, no one has pinpointed a single culprit.

Many viruses have been implicated. The Herpes family of viruses has received the most scrutiny. As viruses go, they tend to be on the large side. They also differ from most other viruses in that their genes contain DNA—just like animal cells. Other viruses contain RNA which is the genetic material found in plant cells. Herpes viruses have the ability to hide inside various body cells in a dormant state ready to emerge and infect at an opportune moment. The word "herpes" brings to mind visions of painful eruptions on the mouth and genitals. Oral and genital Herpes are caused by Herpes Simplex viruses (HSV). HSV-1 causes oral Herpes. HSV-2 infects the genitals. However, Herpes contains many more family members than Simplex one and two. Herpes also includes the Varicella-zoster virus (the cause of chicken pox and shingles) and the group of viruses that are presumed to cause CFS: Epstein-Barr virus (EBV), Cytomegalovirus (CMV) and the Herpes - 6 virus or (HHV6).

EPSTEIN-BARR VIRUS (EBV), ORIGIN

In 1985, reports were published in the *Annals of Internal Medicine* about a mysterious severe viral epidemic that gripped the Lake Tahoe region in California. In retrospect, those reports were the entré of CFS into public consciousness. Initially, CFS was presumed to be caused by the Epstein-Barr Virus because research at the National Institutes of Health confirmed the presence of elevated levels of antibodies against EBV in afflicted people. As time passed, however, EBV was deemed to be one of many viruses associated with the CFS syndrome *as a result of the disease, but not as a primary cause.* Even so, these other viral players may have a profound effect on the total symptom picture of CFS, though they are just passengers on a vehicle that is being driven by a mysterious virus.

In trying to comprehend the vast panorama of symptoms that occur in CFS, it is helpful to get a good view of the individual agents that comprise the disease. Let us begin with EBV. We know that EBV causes the debilitating disease of teenhood,"Infectious Mononucleosis," or, in lay parlance, 'mono' (sometimes called 'the kissing disease'). But, not everyone who carries this virus develops 'mono'. In fact, over 90% of Americans have been exposed to EBV by age 20, and only a small fraction of these people become laid up.

The consequences of primary (first) exposure are variable. Some patients develop infectious mononucleosis; others simply experience flu-like symptoms for a few days, and most show no symptoms at all. Like all herpes viruses, however, EBV remains in the body for life. This is normally of little consequence, as an individual's immune system usually keeps the virus in a latent or inactive state.

It is now known, however, that latent EBV can be reactivated into a chronic (persistent) infection. How and when this happens depends upon a number of factors, most prominent being the strength of the individual's immune system. Stephen Straus, a leading virologist and EBV researcher, has stated that the reservoir of latent EBV virus acts as a "barometer of immunocompetence," and concludes that chronic illness is often "an indicator of faulty immune containment of EBV."

It is clear, for example, that when the immune system is suppressed, EBV often flares up. It is not surprising then to find EBV on the list of "opportunistic infections" commonly affecting AIDS and cancer patients. Similarly, one of the most serious risks for organ transplant patients is EBV infection, since there is a critical period during which immunosuppressive drugs are used to prevent rejection of the foreign tissue. Aside from these obvious cases, EBV can affect individuals whose immune systems have been weakened by a variety of factors. *Conditions which contribute to this process include surgery, emotional stress, allergies, exposure to environmental toxins, and a genetic predisposition.*

In addition, a number of illnesses have been identified that appear to be involved with Epstein-Barr virus activity, including other viral illnesses, rheumatoid arthritis, malaria, intestinal parasites and recurrent candida yeast infection.

How is EBV related to mononucleosis?

Infectious mononucleosis is a condition marked by debilitating fatigue, fever, sore throat, and swollen lymph glands. It is caused by the Epstein-Barr virus, and usually lasts from 3 to 6 weeks. It is interesting to note that mononucleosis is rare in lesser developed and in overcrowded regions of the world, where children are quickly exposed to the Epstein-Barr virus. On the other hand, in the materially privileged Western world, contact with EBV often does not take place until adolescence. About half the time, this delayed exposure leads to infectious mononucleosis.[1]

Until recently, it was thought that mononucleosis patients produced sufficient antibodies to keep them immune from future EBV infection. In light of current research, however, this picture has been changed. It is now believed that individuals who have had mononucleosis are slightly more susceptible to recurrent EBV than the general population.[2] Is EBV contagious? Yes and No. Yes, it is easy to expose oneself to EBV because it can be transmitted via saliva. This is why the virus is said to be so common in man. On the other hand, when we speak of a contagious virus, we usually mean the active debilitating stage of illness. In this sense, EBV is not easily communicable, as is for example the common cold. Individuals in close contact with EBV patients, in fact, do not seem to develop EBV infection any more frequently than the general population.[3] The same holds true for families where one member has acute infectious mononucleosis.[4]

Recently, immunologists conducted a long-term study with 54 married women in their mid to late 20's, all of whom had tested negative for EBV. The researchers were interested to find that over the course of a year, only one woman was infected with the virus. What was more surprising, however, was the fact that two of these women were married to men with active EBV infections and still did not become infected themselves. The researchers concluded that intimate exposure to the virus by adults does not necessarily result in infection.[5] The key, as we have said, is to establish and maintain a powerful and vigilant immune system.

How is EBV related to CFS? Physicians and researchers began to recognize the incidence of recurrent mononucleosis as early as 1948.[6] Reports continued to appear throughout the 50's and 60's[7-10], but it wasn't until the late 1970's that studies were published describing the occurrence of persistent and long-term EBV infection characterized by intermittent fever, muscle and joint aches, sore throats, and debilitating fatigue.[11,12] Unlike mononucleosis, this condition did not seem to be self limiting. It would come and go, or never fully abate. Patients described it as a perpetual flu, a feeling of physical and mental exhaustion. In the mid 1980's, numerous studies were published which seemed to correlate these symptoms directly with reactivation of latent EBV.[13-16] This disorder was therefore referred to as chronic Epstein-Barr virus syndrome, or CEBV. Symptoms varied, but usually included extreme fatigue, weakness, depression, muscle and joint aches, sore throat, swollen lymph glands, headache and low-grade afternoon fever. In addition, many patients reported impaired memory, difficulty concentrating, disturbed balance, anxiety, irritability and insomnia. These symptoms usually fluctuated in severity from month to month, and even day to day. Unfortunately, periods of wellness were often followed by relapse, as patients attempted to resume normal activities or strenuous exercise.

We began compiling research and clinical data on our CEBV patients in 1985. Gradually, a pattern of illness began to emerge which included more than just EBV. We therefore began talking about a syndrome in which EBV was perhaps the major, but certainly not the only factor. It was also possible, we reasoned, that EBV was being reactivated due to a weakness in immune function, and that this weakness could have a number of causes. This is difficult for some patients and doctors to understand. People are so used to a single-cause mechanism for diseases that they miss the importance of a multifactorial syndrome. Influenza virus causes flu, herpes simplex causes herpes, and because EBV causes mononucleosis (characterized by chronic fatigue) it was natural to believe that EBV alone caused Chronic Fatigue Syndrome. We disagreed.

Late in 1987, research began to appear which supported our view. A surprisingly high percentage of individuals (20% to 24% in general medical practices) were found to be suffering from this specific group of symptoms.[17-19] It became apparent, however, that other disorders had to be involved in the syndrome because the severity of Epstein-Barr virus varied widely from patient to patient.

Unfortunately, this has caused some clinicians to conclude that EBV has nothing to do with chronic fatigue. Others now claim that Chronic Epstein-Barr virus is impossible to diagnose. Nothing could be further from the truth. It is only accurate to say that additional factors besides Epstein-Barr virus must be explored, and that the name of the disorder should reflect the wider definition. Thus the term in present use is *Chronic Fatigue and Immune Dysfunction Syndrome*. As we have said, we prefer the shorter and simpler CFS.

MORE UNWANTED GUESTS

CYTOMEGALOVIRUS (CMV)

Although not as common as EBV, CMV is estimated to infect close to 75% of adults in Western nations, with the incidence in Asia and Africa approaching 100%.[20,21] In the majority of cases, primary exposure produces no clinical illness, but like all herpes viruses, CMV remains latent in the body for life. During times of immune suppression, CMV can become reactivated and produce symptoms very similar to EBV. In fact, 10 to 15% of all mononucleosis cases appear to be caused by CMV and not EBV.[22] For the most part, however, CMV produces observable illness in two groups: infants and immune suppressed adults. Every year, millions of babies worldwide are born with congenital CMV infections. In lesser-developed nations where poverty, disease (especially malaria), and malnutrition are common, 10 to 20% of children are infected.[23] In contrast to this dismal scenario, the frequency of infection in the U.S. ranges from 1% to 3%.[24] The consequences of congenital infection vary. Fortunately, most children "take it in stride" and manifest no overt disease. About 10 to 20% of infected infants (3 to 5 out of every thousand births), however, will develop serious illness, often resulting in brain and central nervous system damage. CMV, in fact, is known to be the major cause of sensory-motor retardation.[25] In addition, about 17% of infected infants who are free of symptoms at birth may develop subsequent hearing impairment or respiratory illness within the first year of life.[26] Obviously, pre-term infants are at high risk due to their under-developed immune systems. How are infants exposed to CMV? Infection takes place in utero when virus passes from the mother to the developing fetus. Children may also be exposed to infectious virus in the birth canal. The severity and duration of infection appear to be dependent on a large number of variables which are not well understood, including the stage of fetal development when exposure occurs.

Other aspects of the CMV virus are equally mysterious. Women who have been exposed to CMV (most women of childbearing age) will have antibodies against the virus, but that does not prevent fetal or neo-natal infection of their children. These neutralizing antibodies, however, are also passed to the new-born in breastmilk, and may play a role in overcoming infection after birth.

It is also highly unlikely that an anti-CMV drug will be developed that is safe for pregnant women. Since that eliminates the major avenue of viral control, it would appear that nothing can be done to eradicate CMV. We believe, however, that taking care of the mother minimizes any risk to the baby. It is important to make sure she is optimally nourished and reduce as much as possible the numerous factors which promote viral activity. All of this is discussed in Chapter 9. Is there any objective support for such a program? Absolutely. It is no coincidence that nations which have the most extensive prenatal care systems, including nutritional support, have the lowest incidence of congenital CMV infection.

In Scandanavia, for example, less than one in 250 children is born with CMV, and of that group, less than 10% develop serious illness from the infection.[27] Prevailing medical opinion today is that CMV infection in adults is uneventful except in cases of organ transplant, transfusion, or immune suppression. Let's look at this. Organ transplant recipients face a triple danger from CMV. Seronegative patients (those with no previous CMV exposure) are often infected by the transplanted tissue. Since the kidney is a major site of CMV infection,[28] it is not surprising to find that kidney transplant operations result in CMV infection in more than 90% of cases.[29] Most transplant patients also undergo transfusion which increases risk to CMV infection from the donor's blood. Remember that the majority of adults have been exposed to CMV before age 30. Even if they have never experienced any illness connected with this exposure, the CMV virus remains in a dormant or latent state. These seropositive patients also risk serious CMV disease when undergoing transplant operations because the stress of surgery and immunosuppressive drug therapy tend to reactivate latent infections. When all is said and done, *researchers agree that CMV is the major factor determining the success or failure of organ transplant operations.*[30]

Also at risk, in addition to transfusion and organ transplant recipients, are those whose immune systems have been damaged by diseases such as AIDS, cancer or leukemia. Once again, it is not surprising to find that CMV infection is almost universal in patients with AIDS or AIDS related complex (ARC). Research shows, in fact, that this disease connection is a vicious cycle that runs in both directions. The AIDS virus depletes the body's T-cell immune system which then allows resident viruses like EBV and CMV to become active. Active CMV and EBV infections, in turn, accelerate the progression of AIDS.[31-33] There are, thus, two distinct groups of people who are most vulnerable to CMV infection. At one end of the spectrum are infants exposed to the virus. At the other end are adults with cancer or AIDS, and patients receiving organ transplants, transfusions and immunosuppressive drugs. What about the rest of us; the vast majority of American adults represented by the area between these two points? According to conservative medical opinion, lifelong CMV infection in the normal individual is considered to be entirely benign. One infectious disease specialist has identified dramatic alterations of immune chemistry due to CMV infection. Yet because there is no outwardly observable symptom related to these events, he asserts that latent infection is of no immunological consequence.[34] We believe that such a conclusion is unsound. The lack of overt CMV disease (i.e. CMV mononucleosis) does not eliminate the possibility that CMV may be a factor in other illnesses. In fact, ever since the late 1970's, evidence has been accumulating which shows that CMV can be involved with a number of health disorders in the "normal" individual. We know, for example, that CMV can infect a wide variety of tissues, including internal organs such as the lung, kidney and liver. It has been estimated that the virus contributes to over 70% of chronic renal (kidney) failure.[35] Likewise, CMV infection of the pancreas has led many investigators to include the virus as a possible causative agent in both juvenile and adult-onset diabetes.[36,37] Animal and human studies show conclusively that CMV and EBV can weaken immunity in the lungs, opening the door to a number of respiratory disorders.[38-41] In addition, CMV and EBV can both infect the central nervous system in adults, causing a wide range of neurologic symptoms ranging from confusion and memory loss to inflammation of the brain (encephalitis),[42,43] and a common nervous system disorder known as Guillain-Barré Syndrome.[44,45] CMV is known to infect the gastrointestinal tract.[46] Once again, this is considered to be a common, and therefore normal occurance. Current research, however, suggests that the virus may contribute to ulcers,[47] colitis,[48] and even cancer of the colon.[49] Other types of cancer have also been associated with CMV. CMV does not cause cancer, but there is at this point no doubt that, like EBV, the virus contributes directly to a number of pre-malignant and malignant disorders.[50-53]

We believe that the job of medical researchers is to look beyond the narrow single-cause model of disease. Fifty years ago, researchers recognized that viruses often act in concert with other pathogens in causing disease.[54] Why are so many of today's clinicians ignoring this fact? There are many factors which allow common viruses like EBV and CMV to tip the immunological balance in favor of disease. Only when these factors are known, can one ever hope to practice preventive health care, or deal successfully with the Chronic Fatigue Syndrome.

RELATIONSHIP of CMV to the CHRONIC FATIGUE SYNDROME

The fundamental point of this book is that persistent illness contributes in specific and predictable ways to a vicious cycle in which immunity is impaired and serious illness results. We will describe how this illness taxes the body's hormone, enzyme and energy reserves, leading directly to chronic fatigue. The herpes viruses, especially EBV and CMV, are important elements in this scenario. Other "resident pathogens" will be introduced in Chapter 6.

Is CMV a common problem? Considering the number of congenitally infected infants and the increasing incidence of CMV-related disease in adults, one leading virologist has concluded, *"The cumulative antisocial consequences of cytomegalovirus infection are massive in degree and impinge on all members of our society."*[55] Those who continue to view these viral infections as benign are like fire fighters who ignore billowing smoke on the horizon, responding only to the blaze, the discovery of which inevitably follows. Such attitudes are still prevalent today, illustrated by a common error in chronic fatigue research. Numerous studies have been reported where Chronic Fatigue Syndrome (CFS) patients were evaluated for EBV. When the researchers found no consistent elevation of EBV antibody levels, they concluded that viruses do not play a role in CFS.[56,57] Other clinicians then cite such "evidence" and conclude that CFS is therefore a psychosomatic disorder—that all of these patients are really suffering from depression.[58] What's wrong with this picture? First of all, the fact that CFS patients tend to be depressed should not lead one to conclude that chronic fatigue is an emotional disorder. More than likely, it is the chronic fatigue that is creating the depression! Secondly, EBV is not the only possible viral agent in chronic fatigue, but very few researchers have bothered to evaluate the presence of CMV orther viruses. Recent studies have shown, however, that CMV growth in the blood can increase significantly long before the onset of clinical symptoms,[59] and that 10% to 15% of all mononucleosis cases are caused by CMV, not EBV.[60] In addition, chronic, debilitating fatigue has been associated with CMV,[61] as well as a combination of CMV and EBV.[62] *Moreover, when researchers include CMV, EBV and Herpes simplex in their evaluations, Chronic Fatigue Syndrome patients are found to have significantly higher viral antibody levels than healthy controls.*[63,64] This should not surprise anyone familiar with viruses. It is well known that there is a close genetic and immunologic relationship, including cross reactivity, between most members of the herpes virus family.[65-67]

Thus current research supports the concept of Chronic Fatigue Syndrome as a multifactorial disorder in which a number of pathogens play significant roles: a condition, in other words, resulting from cumulative immune stress in which the presence of one resident virus may directly enhance the proliferation of a second. EBV, for example is kept under control by Immune T-cells, but these T-cells can be infected and destroyed by other viruses. The most well known

T-cell virus is the HIV or AIDS virus, and HIV infection usually leads to EBV disease.[68] In addition, a certainly less serious but more prevalent synergy may exist between members of the herpes virus family, as both CMV and HHV-6 have both been found to infect T-cells.[69-71]

In summary, both CMV and EBV contribute to the Chronic Fatigue Syndrome. Research shows, however, that EBV tends to be more common and more virulent. In the following chapters, therefore, we will speak primarily of EBV, understanding that CMV is closely related and often present. Fortunately, both viruses are treated in the same way. Both can be controlled via anti-viral therapy and immune building techniques. (see Chapter 1). In our clinical practice, for example, recovery is characterized by decreasing antibody levels for all the herpes viruses, along with diminished symptoms and increased energy.

HUMAN HERPESVIRUS TYPE 6 (HHV-6)

In October, 1986, researchers from the National Cancer Institute reported the discovery of a new human virus. Since it infected B-lymphocyte cells, they named the virus Human B Lymphotropic Virus (HBLV).[72] Further research identified the new virus as a herpesvirus,[73] and because it was also found to infect other cells including T-cells, the name was changed to human herpesvirus type 6 (HHV-6).

How is HHV-6 related to Chronic Fatigue Syndrome? It is still too early to know if and how this new virus is involved in CFS. Since blood tests for HHV-6 have only recently become available to clinical physicians, we have to rely on research data for information. Here is what we know: HHV-6 was first identified in patients with AIDS and other serious immune disorders. HHV-6 has been identified as a primary cause of some cases of teenage mononucleosis. When a number of CFS patients from the Lake Tahoe area also tested positive, some lay health writers jumped to the conclusion that HHV-6 causes Chronic Fatigue Syndrome. This has proven not to be the case, although medical researchers are presently considering that HHV-6 may be one "trigger" which turns on EBV and other viruses.

It is becoming evident that almost 90% of Americans have been exposed to the Herpes 6 virus in infancy.[74] However, illness from Herpes 6 is rare and blood antibody levels remain low in the vast majority of the normal population. In Chronic Fatigue Syndrome patients, the frequency of active infection appears to be closer to 60%.[75,76] If this scenario sounds familiar, it is because we have gone through it before in our discussion of EBV and CMV. HHV-6 is most likely a rather common herpesvirus. Once an individual is exposed, the virus remains in a latent or dormant state for life. When immunity is impaired, as in AIDS and cancer patients, the virus can proliferate to detectable levels.

Chronic Fatigue Syndrome, as we will describe, is a phenomena resulting not from one virus, but from a group of disease stressors which weaken immunity. We are not surprised at all by the finding that CFS patients have higher than normal levels of HHV-6 antibodies. It is well known that most CFS patients have higher than normal levels of antibodies to the entire herpesvirus family.[77] Current research also shows that as many as 50% of CFS patients harbor enterovirus infections such as Coxsackie virus.[78] One cannot, therefore, say that EBV, CMV, herpes simplex or HHV-6 alone causes Chronic Fatigue Syndrome. Instead, they are associated with the disorder in a chicken-and-egg relationship described in detail in Chapter 6.

Examining a failing business, financial experts will look for production, personnel, and cash flow problems, as well as sales and marketing errors. They will not, however, quibble about which came first. Likewise, with Chronic Fatigue, we believe that it makes more sense to identify and treat all disease factors, and at the same time work to strengthen the immune system. Today, HHV-6 is an "orphan virus" with no specific clinical symptoms associated with infection. Two recent findings, however, suggest that the virus may play a role in the progression of AIDS and certain types of cancer.[79,80]

Whether HHV-6 turns out to be a virulent and destructive pathogen or "just another herpes virus," it will probably be vulnerable to the same anti-viral and immune-stimulating therapies that we describe in Chapter 10. If you are looking for a simple vaccine or a miracle cure, our approach will disappoint you. Defending yourself from viruses and other pathogens is not an easy task. The good news, of course, is that it can be done, and there are clear guidelines to recovery from what was once thought to be a hopeless condition.

THE RETROVIRUS CONNECTION

In September, 1990, a stunning presentation was delivered to an international scientific conference in Japan which confirmed the presence of a retrovirus in CFS patients. Retrovirus rumors had been circulating for almost two years and had staggering implications. If such a virus existed, it would link CFS with the same class of viruses responsible for several types of leukemia and AIDS!

Retroviruses have only been identified as causes of human disease for the past decade. They have all been given the prefix 'HTLV' which stands for "Human T Cell Leukemia" virus.

HTLV 1 has been identified as the cause of Human T Cell Leukemia and was discovered in 1980.

HTLV 2 has been identified as the cause of Hairy Cell Leukemia and was discovered in 1982.

HTLV 3 was an early name for the virus that causes AIDS and was discovered in 1986.

The potential CFS retrovirus, actually appears to closely resemble HTLV 2 and may be a mutant strain of that virus.

At this symposium, Dr. Elaine De Freitas of the Wistar Institute in Philadelphia reported the presence of this new retrovirus in the white blood cells of 75% of the CFS patients who were studied. In contrast this virus was not present at all in healthy normal people who served as controls. Perhaps even more startling was the identification of this virus in one third of people who were casual contacts of CFS patients but who did not necessarily have CFS themselves. These non-sexual contacts could have been the playmates of afflicted children or the co-workers of sick adults.

This last finding was a big surprise. Retroviruses have not been suspected of spreading by casual contact but only through blood, semen or breast milk. Could this be a special strain of an exceptionally contagious retrovirus? Could this casual contagion help to explain the occurrence of CFS epidemics afflicting entire communities?

Not so fast! The "Wistar" virus was only found to *exist* in CFS patients. It has not yet been established as a cause of the disease. The Herpes 6 virus has also been found in about 75% of CFS patients and yet is thought to be only an accessory to a crime perpetrated by an as yet unidentified virus.[81]

However, exciting confirmation of the retrovirus theory occurred in September, 1991 with widely publicized reports that a "spumavirus" was detected in the spinal fluid of 50% of CFS patients by Dr. John Martin, a pathologist at the University of Southern California School of Medicine. It was surmised that the spumavirus—which is also a retrovirus—may be identical to the Wistar strain discovered by Dr. De Freitas.

REFERENCES

1. Henle G. Henle W. The virus as the etiologic agent of infectious mononucleosis. In: Epstein, M.A., Achong, B.G. (eds.) *The Epstein-Barr Virus*. New York: Springer-Verlag, 1979.
2. DuBois RE, Seeley JK, *et al.* Chronic mononucleosis syndrome. *Southern Med J.*, 1984; 77(11):1376-1382.
3. Fleisher, G.R., Pasquariello, P.S., Warren, W.S., *et al.* Intrafamilial transmission of Epstein-Barr virus infection. *J Pediat.*, 1981; 98:16-19.
4. Wahren, B, Lantorp K, Sterner G, Espmark A: EBV antibodies in family contacts of patients with infectious mononucleosis. *Proc Soc Exper Biol Med.*, 1970; 133:934-939.
5. Chang, R.S., Le, C.T. Failure to acquire Epstein-Barr virus infection after intimate exposure to the virus. *Am J Epidemiol.*, 1984; 119(3):392-5.
6. Isaacs, R. Chronic infectious mononucleosis. *Blood*, 1948; 3:858.
7. Kaufman, R.E. Recurrences in infectious mononucleosis. *Am Pract.*, 1950; 1:673.
8. Patterson, J.K., Pinninger, J.L. Recurrent infectious mononucleosis. *Br Med J.*, 1955; 2:476.
9. Bender, C.E. Recurrent mononucleosis. *JAMA* 1962; 182:954.
10. Graves, S. Jr., Recurrent infectious mononucleosis. *J Ky Med Assoc.*, 1970; 1:790.
11. Smith, H. Denman AM: A new manifestation of infection with Epstein-Barr virus. *Br Med J Clin Res.*, 1978; 2:248.
12. Fry, J. Infectious mononucleosis: Some new observations from a 15 year study. *J Fam Pract.*, 1980; 10: 1087.
13. Jones, J.F., Ray, C.G., *et al.* Evidence for active Epstein-Barr virus infection in patients with persistent, unexplained illnesses: elevated anti-early antigen antibodies. *Ann Int Med.*, 1985; 102(1):1-6.
14. Straus, S.E., Tosato, G., *et al.* Persisting illness and fatigue in adults with evidence of Epstein-Bar virus infection. *Ann Int Med.*, 1985; 102: 7-16.
15. J. Tobi, M., Morag, A., Ravid, Z. *et al.* Prolonged atypical illness associated with serological evidence of persistent Epstein-Barr virus infection. *Lancet*, 1982; 1:61.
16. DuBois, R.E., Seeley, J.K., *et al.* Chronic mononucleosis syndrome. *South Med J.*, 1984; 77:1376.
17. Holmes, G.P., Kaplan, J.E., *et al.* A cluster of patients with a chronic mononucleosis-like syndrome: is Epstein-Barr virus the cause? *JAMA*, 1987; 257:2297.
18. Buchwald, D., Sullivan, J.L., Komaroff, A.L. Frequency of "chronic active Epstein-Barr virus infection" in a general medical practice. *JAMA*, 1987; 257:2303.
19. Kroenke, K., Wood, D.R., Mangelsdorff, A.D., Meier, N.J., Powell, J.B. Chronic fatigue in primary care; Prevalence, patient characteristics and outcome. *JAMA*, 1988; 260(7):929.
20. Stern, H., Elek, S.D. The incidence of infection with cytomegalovirus in a normal population- a serological study in greater London. *J Hyg.*, 1965; 63:79.
21. Krech, U.H., Jung, M., Jung, F. *Cytomegalovirus Infections of Man*, Basel, S. Karger Publishers, 1971.
22. Hamilton, J.D. Cytomegalovirus and immunity. *Monographs in Virology*, 1982; vol 12.
23. Reynolds, D.W., *et al. New Eng J Med.*, 1973; 289:1.

24. Doerr, H.W. Cytomegalovirus infection in pregnancy. *J Environ Methods.*, 1987; 17(1-2):127.

25. Stagno, S., Reynolds, D.W., *et al.* Congenital cytomegalovirus infection—occurrence in an immune population. *New Eng J Med.*, 1977; 296:1254.

26. Stagno, S., Reynolds, D.W., *et al. Pediatrics.* 1977; 59:669.

27. Ahlfors, K., *et al. Scand J Infect Dis.*, 1979; 11:177.

28. Heieren, M.H., van der Woude, F.J., Balfour, H.H. Jr. Cytomegalovirus replicates efficiently in human mesangial cells. *Proc Natl Acad Sci (USA)*, 1988; 85:1642.

29. Fiala, M., Payne, J.E., *et al.* Epidemiology of cytomegalovirus infection after transplantation and immunosuppression. *J Infect Dis.*, 1975; 132:421.

30. Rubin, R.H., Russell, P.V., Levin, M. Cohen, C. *J Infect Dis.*, 1979; 139:728.

31. Rando, R.F., Pellett, P.E., *et al.* Transactivation of human immunodeficiency virus by herpes viruses. *Oncogene*, 1987; 1:13.

32. Skolnik, P.R., Kosloff, B.R., Hirsch, M.S. Bidirectional interactions between human immunodeficiency virus type 1 and cytomegalovirus. *J Infect Dis.*, 1988; 157: 508.

33. Safai, B., Lynfield, R., Lowenthal, D.A., Koziner, B. Cancers associated with HIV infection. *Anticancer Res.*, 1987; 7:1055.

34. Hamilton, J.D. Cytomegalovirus and immunity. *Monographs in Virology*, 1982; vol 12.

35. Spencer, E.S., Cytomegalovirus antibody in uremic patients prior to renal transplantation. *Scand J Infect Dis.*, 1974; 6.

36. Craighead, J.E. *Acta Endocrinol.*, 1976; 83(Suppl 205):123.

37. Ward, K.P., Galloway, W.H., Auchterlonie, I.A. *Lancet*, 1979; 1:497.

38. Shanley, J.D., Pesanti, E.L. Replication of murine cytomegalovirus in lung macrophages: effect on phagocytosis of bacteria. *Infect Immunity*, 1980; 29:1152.

39. Reynolds, H.Y. Host defense impairments that may lead to respiratory infections. *Clin Chest Med.*, 1987; 8(3):339.

40. Luby, J.P. Pneumonias in adults due to mycoplasma, chlamydiae, and viruses. *Am J Med Sci.*, 1987; 294(1):45.

41. Andiman, W.A., McCarthy, P., *et al.* Clinical, virologic and serologic evidence of Epstein-Barr virus infection in association with childhood pneumonia. *J Pediatr.*, 1981; 99:880.

42. Phillips, C.A., Fanning, W.L., Gump, D.W., Phillips, C.F. Cytomegalovirus encephalitis in immunologically normal adults. Successful treatment with vidarabine. *JAMA*, 1977; 28:2299.

43. Schiff, J.A., Schaefer, J.A., Robinson, J.E. Epstein-Barr virus incerebrospinal fluid during infectious mononucleosis encephalitis. *Yale J Biol Med.*, 1982; 55:59.

44. Schmitz, H., Enders, G. Cytomegalovirus as a frequent cause of Guillain-Barre' Syndrome. *J Med Virol.*, 1977; 1:21.

45. Glaser, R., Brennan, R., Berlin, C.M. Guillain-Barre' syndrome associated with Epstein-Barr virus in a cytomegalovirus-negative patient. *Dev Med Child Neurol.*, 1981; 38:134.

46. Weller, T.H. *New Eng J Med.*, 1971; 285:203.

47. Campbell, D.A., Piercey, J.R.A., *et al. Gastroenterology*, 1977; 72:533.

48. Keren, D.F., Milligan, F.D., *et al. Johns Hopkins Med J.*, 1975; 136:178.

49. Roche, J.K., Huang, E-S. *Gastroenterology*, 1977; 72:228.

50. Koop, H.O., Holodniy M., List, A.F. Fulminant Kaposi's sarcoma complicating long-term corticosteroid therapy. *Am J Med.*, 1987; 787.

51. Macnab, J.C. Herpes simplex virus and human cytomegalovirus: their role in morphological transformation and genital cancers. *J Gen Virol.*, 1987; 68(Pt 10):2525.

52. Rapp, F. Cytomegalovirus and carcinogenesis. *JNCI*, 1984;

53. Giraldo, G., Beth, E., Huang, E.S. Kaposi's sarcoma and its relationship to cytomegalovirus (CMV): 3. CMV DNA and CMV early antigens in Kaposi's sarcoma. *Int J Cancer*, 1980; 26:23.

54. Rivers, T. Viruses and Koch's postulates. *J Bacteriol.*, 1937;33:1

55. Weller, T.H. Clinical spectrum of cytomegalovirus infection. In: A.J. Nahmias, W.R. Dowdle, R.F. Schinazi (eds.) *The Human Herpesviruses*, New York, Elsevier, 1981.

56. Chronic Fatigue: Epstein-Barr virus connection disputed. *Med World News*, 1988; 29(11):35.

57. Buchwald, D., Sullivan, J.L., Komaroff, A.L. Frequency of chronic active Epstein-Barr virus infection in a general medical practice. *JAMA* 1987; 257(17):2303.

58. Jacobson, E.J. Chronic mononucleosis: it almost never happens. *Postgrad Med.*, 1988; 83(1):56.

59. Spector, S., Rina, J., Spector, D., McMillan, R. *J Infect Dis* ., 1984; 150:121.

60. Hamilton, J.D. Cytomegalovirus and immunity. *Monographs in Virology*, 1982; vol 12.

61. Pether, J.V.S., Isaac, D.H., Penny, P.T. *Br Med J.*, 1978; 1:597 ---Weller, T.H. The cytomegaloviruses: ubiquitous agents with protean clinical manifestations. *New Eng J Med.*, 1971; 285:203 &267.

62. Lemon, S.M., Hutt, L.M., *et al. Am J Med.*, 1979; 66:270.

63. Holmes, G.P., Kaplan, J.E., *et al.* A cluster of patients with a chronic mononucleosis-like syndrome. Is Epstein-Barr virus the cause? *JAMA*, 1987; 257(17):2297.

64. Straus, S.E., Dale, J.K., *et al.* Acyclovir treatment of the chronic fatigue syndrome: lack of efficacy in a placebo-controlled trial. *New Eng J Med.*, 1988; 319(26):1692.

65. Cranage, M.P., Smith, G.L., *et al.* Identification and expression of a human cytomegalovirus glycoprotein with homology to the Epstein-Barr virus BXLF2 product, varicella-zoster virus gpIII, and herpes simplex virus type 1 glycoprotein H. *J Virol.* 1988; 62(4):1416.

66. Anders, D.G., Gibson, W. Location, transcript analysis, and partial nucleotide sequence of the cytomegalovirus gene encoding an early DNA-binding protein with similarities to ICP8 of herpes simplex virus type 1. *J Virol.*, 1988 62(4):1364.

67. Balachandran, N., Oba D.E., Hutt-Fletcher, L.M. Antigenic cross-reactions among herpes simplex virus types 1 and 2, Epstein-Barr virus and cytomegalovirus. *J Virology*, 1987; 61(4):1125.

68. Yarchoan R., Redfield R.R., Broder S. Mechanisms of B cell activation in patients with acquired immunodeficiency syndrome and related disorders. Contribution of antibody-producing B cells, and of immunoglobulin production induced by human T cell lymphotropic virus, type III lymphadenopathy-associated virus. *J Clin Invest.*, 1986; 78(2):439.

69. Garnett, H.M. Isolation of human cytomegalovirus from peripheral blood T cells or renal transplant patients. *J Lab Clin Med.*, 1982; 99:92.

70. Schrier, R.D., Nilson, J.A., Oldstone, M.B.A. Detection of human cytomegalovirus in peripheral blood lymphocytes in natural infection. *Science*, 1985; 230:1048.

71. Ablashi, D.V., Salahuddin, S.Z., *et al.* HBLV (or HHV-6) in humanc ell lines. [letter] *Nature*, 1987; 329:207.

72. Salahuddin, S.Z., Ablashi, D.V., *et al.* Isolation of a new virus, HBLV, in patients with lymphoproliferative disorders. *Science*, 1986; 234(4776):596.

73. Biberfeld, P., Kramarsky, B., Salahuddin, S.Z., Gallo, R.C. Ultrastructural characterization of a new human B lymphotropic DNA virus (human herpesvirus 6) isolated from patients with lymphoproliferative disease. *JNCI*, 1987; 79:933.

74. Ablashi, D.V., Salahuddin, S.Z., Kaplan, M., *et al.* Presence of human B-lymphotropic virus (HBLV) antibody in sera from infected AIDS patients. Presented at Third International Congress on AIDS, Washington D.C., June, 1987.

75. Dale, J.K., *et al.* The Inoue-Melnick virus, human herpesvirus Type 6, and the chronic fatigue syndrome. *Ann Int Med.*, 1989; 110-92.

76. Straus, S.E. The chronic mononucleosis syndrome. *J Infect Dis.*, 1988; 157:405

77. Holmes, G.P., Kaplan, J.E., *et al.* A cluster of patients with a chronic mononucleosis-like syndrome. Is Epstein-Barr virus the cause? *JAMA*, 1987; 257:2297.

78. Yousef, G.E., Bell, E.J., *et al.* Chronic enterovirus infection in patients with post-viral fatigue syndrome. *Lancet*, 1988; 1:146.

79. Lusso, P., Markham, P.D., *et al. In vitro* cellular tropism of human B-lymphotropic virus (human herpesvirus-6). *J Exp Med.*, 1988; 167(5):1659.

80. Josephs, S.F., Buchbinder, A., *et al.* Detection of human B-lymphotropic virus (human herpesvirus 6) sequences in B cell lymphoma tissues of three patients. *Leukemia*, 1988; 2(3):132.

81. CFIDS Chronicle: Sept., 1990; 1-16.

CHAPTER 4

YEASTS

Antibiotic treatment for acne may be the single greatest contributor to the Chronic Fatigue Syndrome.

Candidiasis infection by *Candida albicans* (C. *albicans*), is often referred to as Candida Hypersenitivity Syndrome (CHS). CHS is still a controversial syndrome, so it requires discussion.

Presently, most of the medical community does not accept that CHS exsits. This forces many doctors to approach the Candida issue in an intolerant way. This might be best illustrated by an incident in which we had to consult a prominent otolaryngologist in reference to a patient suffering from a chronic sinus infection.

We tactfully suggested that the specialist might consider a candida infection as a cause of the infection, since the patient had a history of recurrent vaginal and intestinal infections suggesting CHS. The patient also had fatigue and many of the confusing symptoms that we've described earlier. Somewhat surprisingly, this doctor did not argue or start a tirade about candidiasis, this "fad diagnosis." More surprising, the reason for his acceptance of possible Candidiasis was that he had never heard of this problem. He was fascinated by the description of both the Candida condition and the controversy. Given the information that follows, it is difficult to believe that the majority of doctors still do not recognize candidiasis as a common cause of chronic fatigue and other related symptoms.

Candida yeast is a normal inhabitant of the gastrointestinal tract, especially the esophagous and the colon (large intestine). A number of factors regulate its growth—primarily the presence or absence of friendly bacteria in the GI tract. When something upsets the balance of bacteria and yeast in the colon, the yeast may proliferate, leading to a yeast invasion of various tissues. We define this invasion as an *infection.* When Candida (also called *monilia*) invades the vagina, it causes a yeast infection which is probably similar to that found in the colon, but much more obvious. Most women have, at some time, suffered this problem with symptoms such as redness, swelling, burning, itching and a thick discharge. Candida, moreover, can proliferate in tissues besides the vagina and colon. It can, in dire circumstances, invade the surface of practically every organ in the human body, even leading to systemic septicemia, a highly lethal bloodstream infection commonly referred to as "blood poisoning." That would be the catastrophic candidiasis that occurs in desperately ill patients[1] such as those with terminal cancer or AIDS.[2] In these severe conditions progressive immune suppression allows the opportunistic yeast free reign to proliferate. The Candida problems which involve CFS and MIS are not lethal to people with a CFS picture. Statistically, however, they may be more important since many people suffer debility from it. Candida infections can also travel throughout the GI tract to the stomach and up the esophagus into the mouth. Once in the mouth and on the tongue, candida infections are referred to as *thrush.* Thrush is more commonly seen in infants who have not yet developed sufficient immunity to the Candida pathogen. In adults, however, thrush may indicate a significant immune deficiency. Until the early 1980's, the prevailing belief was that Candida affects humans in only two ways. In the severely immunocompromised patient, it is a life threatening condition. Otherwise, it has been regarded as a nuisance, mainly to women suffering vaginal yeast infections or men with "jock itch." Candida infection is known to be more frequent in diabetics. Many doctors are still not aware that there is a broad continuum of severity associated with candidiasis. At one end of the continuum, for example, *Candida albicans* can proliferate beyond its benign state to an active state in a very short time.[3]

There are three major categories of Candida yeast infection:

1. Commonly recognized and accepted Candida infections, such as vaginitis, thrush, and various candida eczemas (groin, feet, breasts, etc). These Candida infections may relate to CFS and MIS.
2. Hidden Candida infections of the bowel, vagina, and perhaps one or more additional organ systems. This can also lead to the Candida Hypersensitivity Syndrome. These are the most controversial Candida problems currently disputed by most physicians practicing medicine.
3. Septicemia and severe disseminated Candidiasis. This form can be lethal.

Candida overgrowth occurs primarily in the esophagus, colon, and vagina and, perhaps, the small intestine and the stomach. When this Candida produces *endotoxins*, it creates a variety of problems, particularly if the proliferation of the yeast overgrowth increases. The failure to recognize this process is significant and puzzling, since, as early as 1952, researchers demonstrated that mice could be killed by endotoxins obtained from Candida cultures.[4] Others were able to produce a severe rash simply by placing this material on the skin of human volunteers.[5] At the very least, experts have agreed that Candida endotoxins can easily cause irritation and damage to mucosal tissue, allowing for deeper penetration of the organism and eventual access to the bloodstream.[6]

As we have said, *Candida albicans* normally exists as a relatively harmless yeast component of the intestinal flora, but when conditions are altered to favor proliferation of this organism, it can convert to a potentially troubling invasive form, which behaves quite differently. Many candida experts believe that this invasive or *mycelial* form is primarily responsible for Candida-related diseases. In its yeast form, Candida proliferates by non-invasive budding. As a fungus, it grows by sending out root-like shoots called rhizoids or hyphae; these can penetrate the intestinal mucosa.

Penetration of the inner lining of the GI tract opens the door to absorption of endotoxins, and allows the candida organism to colonize in tissue far from the point of fungal entry in immunocompromized patients.[7]

There is disagreement as to whether Candida can actually survive for long periods in the bloodstream. Researchers report that this is possible, but only in critically ill patients whose immune systems are severely impaired.[8] In otherwise healthy individuals, antibodies, immune cells, and anti-fungal enzymes appear to prevent Candida growth in the blood.[9]

Commonly occurring, however, is the absorption of large amounts of endotoxin into the bloodstream, taxing immune function in numerous and well defined ways.[10-14]

The first stage of candida overgrowth involves the spread of the organism beyond its normal boundaries.

Immune suppression can be considered the second stage, which we will learn is biochemically related to the mixed infection syndrome.

The third stage, for which there is ample evidence, is the potentiation of other pathogens such as viruses, parasites, and bacteria.

What causes candida to spread? Injury is one factor which can lower the body's immune suppression of Candida growth. Burn patients, for example, have been found to be particularly susceptible to Candida infections,[15] as would patients undergoing surgery.[16] Aside from such cases, there are other factors which may affect the growth of yeast.

According to some public health experts, Candida overgrowth may affect as many as 20 million Americans.[17] The vast majority of people afflicted by this condition may be totally unaware of its insidiousness. It is not a catastrophic illness like AIDS, but more like a series of events which can lead to such chronic problems as impaired immunity, disruption of normal body chemistry, and the initiation of long term cycles of infection.

Diet plays an important role in this story because yeasts depend on simple carbohydrates. Yeast grows most rapidly on refined sugar.[18] Refined sugar has been shown to impair some aspects of immune function needed to control yeast overgrowth.[19,20] Additionally, other dietary factors have also been implicated in facilitating the proliferation of *Candida albicans*, including: low fiber diets,[21] poor digestive function leading to poor absorption of nutrients (i.e. achlorhydria),[22] and even malnutrition.[23] Certain drugs have also been implicated in the spread of Candida, including: antibiotics,[24] certain steroids,[25] most birth control pills,[26] and even specific tranquilizers.[27]

Finally, we are also beginning to recognize that there is an essential balance between our immune system and resident pathogens. A landmark review published by the American Society for Microbiology concluded that many individuals experience a modest increase in intestinal yeast proliferation at some time in their life. When this happens, some measurable impairment of immunity may occur until the immune system is able to bring the proliferative activity of Candida under control.[28]

Case History

Ms. K. S. came to our office at age 32, feeling like she hadn't been really well since junior high school. She reported a long history of allergies, frequently treated by her doctor with antihistamines and decongestants. As a child, she was prone to earaches and sore throats, and took antibiotics whenever her infection became painful or a fever developed. At age 15, she was treated with antibiotics for mild acne. (Antibiotic treatment for acne may be the single greatest contributor of CFS.) In high school, she developed a psoriasis-like rash which got worse whenever she was under stress. A dermatologist prescribed cortisone cream which helped but did not eliminate the condition. The rash continued as an episodic problem thereafter.

In college, Karen started to fall apart. Academically, she had no problems, but chronic fatigue often prevented her from enjoying the same activities as her friends. She began to feel depressed, often disoriented or "spacey." The school physician said that she was suffering from hypoglycemia, or low blood sugar, and suggested that she carry a candy bar in her purse to munch on between classes.

Soon afterwards, K.S. noticed that her PMS (Premenstrual Syndrome) was getting much worse. She was used to mild cramping, headache and strange food cravings for two or three days each month, but suddenly these symptoms became severe, and started coming a week or even ten days before her period. Finally, she was feeling so crazy and in such pain that she went to her gynecologist, who put her on birth control pills. Initially it helped, but from then on it seemed she had one vaginal yeast infection after another.

K.S. estimated that she had spent thousands of dollars on prescriptions for her yeast infections. One day, in a sudden flash, she saw how crazy this cycle was. Her medicine cabinet was overflowing with vaginal suppositories, cortisone skin creams, antibiotics, antihistamines and sinus medication. Yet, she was always sick; she was constantly fatigued. What she didn't realize was that she had CFS.

In talking with us, she made an important observation, which has been shared by other patients with CFS: that with each drug she took she seemed to have multiple effects. One effect was the intended suppression of her symptom; yet, there always seemed to be "side effects." Sometimes, the "cure" was worse than the disease. She wondered what role her various medications played in her on-going problems. She now wondered what alternatives existed.

We found clinical evidence of yeast infection by blood and stool tests. As a result, she was placed on a treatment regime that consisted of diet management, supplementation of nutrients designed to suppress the proliferative Candida growth, and an antifungal medication called Nystatin. In time, this combination did well for her. In fact, in several months, she seemed fully recovered. Her energy levels reached near normal levels while her skin and vaginal problems disappeared.

K.S., however, was a relatively easy patient to treat. Many others require much more intense treatment, some of which we will describe in greater detail in subsequent chapters.

As far as her experience with side effects from prescription drugs, we would say that most medications produce side effects. We agree with the critics who claim that antibiotics are overused. All too often we are left with no other conclusion but that antibiotic use was somehow initimately involved in the eventual overproliferative activity of *Candida albicans*. For patients this results in the chronic debilitating CFS experienced by K. S. Sometimes, remedies as simple as acidophilus-rich yogurts or an acidophilus supplement resolves this problem. When it doesn't, it is a good idea to seek professional help.

Their value, though we criticize the overuse of antibiotics, should not be ignored. World War II ushered in "The Antibiotic Era" of medicine. Post war baby boomers were the first to grow up during this age of wonder drugs. As with all scientific miracles, however, there slowly appeared both good and bad news.

First the good news: Antibiotics cured a significant number of previoulsy fatal diseases, such as septicemia. Today, bacterial endocarditis (heart infection), tuberculosis, bacterial pneumonia, meningitis, rheumatic fever, diphtheria, typhoid fever, syphilis, and gonorrhea, are just some of the examples of formerly lethal or crippling infections, now largely curable due to antibiotics.

In addition, a number of dread diseases, from cholera to salmonella, are now controllable, including a vast array of serious infections found in the tonsils, sinuses, ears, eyes, throat, or skin. No wonder these drugs were hailed as a panacea for mankind. No wonder doctors as a profession where so proud and mothers whisked their children into the doctor's office for a "shot" at the first sign of a cold. It is no wonder that antibiotics became overused by some practitioners.

Now the bad news: Bacteria are only one of the four major groups of pathogenic microorganisms which can cause diseases. The other three are not responsive to antibacterial drugs. The yeast/fungus group is one of these three. Antibiotics, unfortunately, given all their benefits in many cases, may actually cause or, at least, accelerate a proliferation of yeast growth in humans.[29] We will explain how this happens in a moment.

Now we have a dilemma. Only a small fraction of bacteria actually cause disease. Three trillion bacteria live in the human gut. Humans have a natural symbiotic (beneficial) relationship with hundreds of bacterial strains. They assist in metabolism, the intestinal production of essential vitamins (such as vitamin K and B12), and play a vital role in maintaining a healthy intestinal flora by limiting the growth of yeast organisms and other pathogens. There is, on the other hand, no known beneficial relationship between man and any yeast or fungus. We tolerate these organisms because they are part of our internal and external environment, but their existence in the body is, under normal circumstances, carefully controlled.

Antibiotics often kill many beneficial (symbiotic) bacteria as well as the disease causing (pathogenic) bugs. This elimination of natural controls allows the proliferation of Candida yeast in the intestinal tract.[30]

This is not a new discovery; medical researchers saw this coming as early as 1945, when scientists and clinicians noted the rapid increase in fungal related illness subsequent to the administration of antibiotics [31,32] and sulfa drugs.[33] The problems ensuing from destruction of beneficial bacteria turned out to be only the proverbial iceberg tip. By 1949, research was demonstrating that antibiotics also increase the virulence of Candida infection, meaning that the drug has a potentiating effect on the yeast organism itself.[34] A few years later, this was confirmed by the discovery that antibiotics accelerate the conversion of Candida from its yeast form to the invasive fungal form.[35]

A third cause of enhanced Candida growth is the elimination by antibiotics of bacteria which normally compete with yeast for nutrients.[36] This leaves the food for the yeast. That's feeding your enemy. Compounding this injury from antibiotics, many of these antibiotics also depress the body's normal immune defense against fungal infection.[37,38]

In this light, it is not surprising that the antibiotic era led to a dramatic increase of yeast related problems in American hospitals, [39, 40] not only from widespread use of the drugs, but also because of the immune stress of surgery.[41]

About a decade later, steroid drugs (cortisone and derivatives such as prednisone) came into widespread use, once again hailed as a panacea, once again overused by some, and once again eventually demonstrated to be immune suppressive[42] and Candida enhancing.[43]

We are not implying that antibiotics and steroids should not be used. We certainly use them. Obviously, there are situations where these medications are essential. The key words, however, are "priority" and "balance." We prioritize away from antibiotics when we can do so safely, and we attempt to balance them with supplements or medications which will suppress yeast. Forty years of antibiotic and steroid overuse has brought suffering to millions who then entered a continuing battle against fungal infection. K.S. is only one of millions of patients with a history of frequent, perhaps excessive, and certainly not balanced, antibiotic use. Fortunately, there have always been many physicians, especially in universities, who refuse to prescribe antibiotics unless they have clear laboratory and clinical evidence that they are indicated. When this prevalent yeast problem becomes fully recognized, more physicians will take these safeguards to prevent and reverse yeast infections.

Fever is an interesting footnote. We know that a fever is sometimes our best antibiotic. Bacteria which cause infection, live best at about 97 degrees. A fever is the body's way of weakening the bacteria. The fever is good for the patient, unless it gets out of control. In many cases, fever should not be a reason for antibiotics or aspirin; let the fever fight the infection when it can be done safely. When fever is caused by virus, antibiotics should generally not be used.

In line with such thinking, if one uses antibiotics to treat acne, one should monitor Candida growth, and consider concomitant antiyeast therapy, especially if the patient has a history of yeast infection. This argument is strengthened by the research showing that similar prolonged low dose antibiotic administration in laboratory animals has resulted in a high mortality rate due to fungal infection.[44]

Looking back at K.S.'s medical history, it is reasonable to surmise that early antibiotic use set her up for Candida overgrowth, and this overgrowth was responsible for her psoriasis. Research supports the likelihood of a causal relationship between the two disorders.[45]

It is also likely that long term use of cortisone cream contributed to her Candida infection and may have weakened her immune system; cortisone derivatives clearly increase the risk of infection. This would include yeast. Additionally, although it was not documented to the standards of the medical community, from our experience it would be a fair assumption that a latent viral infection such as EBV was reactivated. The use of candy for "energy" is medically unsound and is a direct stimulus to Candida infection.[46]

The combined effect of EBV and Candida could easily have been responsible for exacerbation of her PMS symptoms. The use of birth control pills as treatment is at best a two edged sword. Birth control pills have been shown to foster Candida growth.[47,48]

Can we reach a verdict? Did her medications have anything to do with the terrible way she felt? Did she have CFS and MIS?

Over the years Karen went to seven different gynecologists. None asked her what she was eating, nor did they think it unusual for a woman to experience recurrent yeast infections for ten years.

Did they not wonder why she kept getting infected by the same organism? In fact, it was published in 1977 that vaginal reinfection comes from Candida overgrowth in the bowel.[49]

It is also possible that some of these physicians believed K.S.'s problem to be a mere nuisance, as they wrote out yet another prescription for antifungal medication. It is now understood, however, that such repeated infection results in significant inhibition of the immune response to Candida organisms throughout the body.[50] Thus, a vicious cycle occurs, wherein intestinal overgrowth causes vaginal infections, which in turn further weakens the immune response to the intestinal overgrowth. And around and around we go.

Stories like Karen's abound in our files and those of our colleagues, and it is time for clinicians to realize that Candida is not always innocuous. In addition to its involvement with EBV, Candida associates with numerous disorders, including urinary tract infections,[51] asthma,[52] respiratory disorders,[53] and chronic hives.[54] Invasive Candida albicans can reach the kidneys, resulting in serious injury. There is an editorial in the *Journal of the American Medical Association* warning that such infection is a risk of antibiotic therapy, even in otherwise healthy people.[55] Candida of such severity is rare, but the subtle variety is rampant.

It is important to note that men can also suffer from Candida overgrowth in the gastrointestinal tract, and serious infection of the male genitourinary tract has been reported.[56]

More physicians today are recommending that patients eat some yogurt during and after a course of antibiotics. Since Lactobacillus acidophilus (yogurt culture) is the primary anti-yeast bacterial strain, the idea is to reinoculate the bowel with this beneficial organism and avoid Candida overgrowth. This step in the right direction is not likely to stop all overgrowth of yeast. By itself, the acidophilus supplements will often not be enough. Most commercial yogurt, in fact, no longer contains Acidophilus, it being replaced with less expensive Thermophilus and Bulgaricus strains which are not known to colonize in the gastrointestinal tract.

A little yogurt, therefore, is not the answer. Furthermore, medications are not our only source of antibiotics. Every day, most of us consume meat and poultry which contain significant amounts of antibiotics. These drugs are fed and injected into animals, not to treat infection, but to promote weight gain by preventing infection in the overcrowded pens.[57]

Antibiotics are fed to dairy cows and later appear in the milk.[58] Livestock use, in fact, accounts for nearly half of the 25 million pounds of antibiotics produced in this country each year.[59] This is a practice which enhances the profits of those food producers while endangering our health. The *American Journal of Public Health* recently reported a study showing that individuals who consumed antibiotic treated poultry were more than twice as likely to contract gastroenteritis than those who had not.[60] Whenever practical, we all, therefore, should consume organic (antibiotic and hormone free) meat and poultry, and increase our use of seafood and vegetarian proteins. Other recommendations for reestablishing healthy intestinal flora and overcoming the adverse effects of drug therapy are in Chapter 10.

How do you know if Candida is a problem?

While we do not recommend self diagnosis, there are definite signs for which to look and bring to the attention of your physician.

1. Recurrent vaginal yeast infections. NOTE: Genital Candida infection is not limited to women. Infection in males is often asymptomatic, but may cause burning and itching near the opening of the penis, as well as urinary tract infection and even kidney disease.[61]
2. Recurrent urinary tract infection.
3. Recurrent or stubborn fungal infections such as athlete's foot, "jock itch" or fungal infections of the cuticle or nail bed.
4. Persistent bloating, discomfort and flatulence after eating; especially after sweets.
5. Chronic constipation or diarrhea.
6. Symptoms worsening on damp days or in moldy places.
7. Lightheaded and "tipsy" after a small amount of beer or wine.
8. Severe fatigue and spacey feeling after meals.
9. History of antibiotic therapy which preceded any of the above side effects *which never fully resolved.*

Diagnosis

Candida, like EBV, lives in the vast majority of people. Simple blood tests, therefore, will show antibodies to this organism. In the early 1980's, microbiologists developed more exact procedures to evaluate the presence and severity of Candida exposure. Even so, final diagnosis is still an enigma. It requires at least careful evaluation of medical history, physical exam, laboratory studies (including stool specimen), and, especially, response to treatment, including a low sugar diet. The most definitive diagnostic test may be the clinical response to nystatin and/or a low sugar diet.

Nystatin is an oral anti-Candida drug which has been in use in various topical and oral forms for over a quarter of a century. It has several distinct and important characteristics:

1. It is not absorbed into the blood stream; it therefore only treats candidiasis locally. If taken orally it treats only the GI tract. If taken vaginally, it treats only the vagina.
2. It is perhaps the most specific drug on the market. It treats no other pathogen of which we know. If a patient responds to Nystatin, the disease is Candidiasis, else the response is placebo.

3. The drug is wonderfully safe. There is no known toxicity. It is safe for pregnant women and newborn babies (the most vulnerable patients when it comes to drug toxicity).

With this knowledge of Nystatin we can make certain deductions about a patient's response. If a patient has symptoms and signs of yeast infection, especially when it is long standing, and that patient clearly responds to nystatin treatment, there is a strong likelihood that the patient was infected with Candida. This is a therapeutic trial. The response helps make the diagnosis

Clinical response is the gold standard.

When we treat the Candida part of an MIS, we often delay the use of Nystatin for one or two months, until the immune system is strengthened. Then, by introducing the Nystatin as a single variable, we can confirm the diagnosis by therapeutic trial. This has two advantages: one, it helps confirm the diagnosis as we just stated, and two, it makes the treatment more effective. If we treat with everything initially, there may be die-off reactions and Nystatin failures, because the patient's immune system was not yet strong enough to tolerate the sudden effect of the Nystatin and to stay healthy after obliterating the Candida.

Nystatin may be specific for Candida albicans but it does have shortcomings. For one, a large percentage of patients feel queazy when they use the high long-term dose of Nystatin that is required and cannot access Candida infestations outside of the belly. Newer drugs like Ketoconazole and Fluconazole penetrate into the bloodstream and destroy yeast throughout the entire body and are more powerful yeast killers than Nystatin. These drugs can cause side effects, particularly to the liver, and must be carefully monitored by a physician. Fluconazole is the most effective of the anti-fungal agents and has the least toxicity.

Case History

Nancy was dismayed. After suffering with urinary tract infections (UTI) on and off for over three years, she was scheduled for surgery to have her urethra dilated. She explained her concern. "My doctor tells me that the opening of my urethra is too small and that causes a backup of urine which leads to infection," she said, "but what puzzles me is how my urethra all of a sudden shrank. I mean I never had this problem before a few years ago. What do you think?"

She made an excellent point. Even if her UTI's were brought about by an abnormality in her urethra, would it not be more reasonable to find what caused the narrowing of that tube rather than simply performing surgery to open it up? Furthermore, if the underlying cause were not addressed, repeated surgery would likely be needed in the future. We agreed to explore alternatives with her, and with her internist's approval, postpone the surgery for 90 days.

Nancy had a history of recurrent vaginal yeast infections and antibiotic use. Since antibiotics foster the growth of Candida in the urinary tract,[62] it was certainly reasonable to consider that a fungal infection might be the cause of obstruction. Since her tests confirmed a considerable overgrowth of Candida in the colon, we decided to initiate anti-fungal therapy.

In addition, Nancy's blood tests showed extreme elevations of IgE antibodies, suggesting that allergy could also be involved. We and others have long been aware that recurrent urinary symptoms can be caused by food and even inhalant allergy.[63, 64]

Results: We began Nancy on a diet and nutritional supplements which resulted in a mild improvement after one month. We then added Nystatin with immediate dramatic improvement. This could be construed as a successful therapeutic trial. After 90 days on the hypoallergenic, low sugar diet and antifungal therapy, Nancy was free of UTI symptoms. After one year of follow up, she told us that when she is under a great deal of stress, or "junks out" on her diet, she still may get a vaginal yeast infection. But if she gets back on her program, the problem is short lived and has never developed into a urinary tract infection.

What can we conclude from all this? Our conclusion about Candida is that it is a major force for illness. It is a frequent contributor to CFS, MIS and of course CHS (Candida Hypersensitivity Syndrome). Furthermore, it is diagnosable and treatable by a number of modalities. The best part is that the treatments often work, and when they do, the patient improves beautifully.

When we tie Candidiasis in with other infections, we get a common version of the MIS. It is commonly seen in association with parasites. In those patients we may then see elevations of their antibody levels as we saw in L.S. in Chapter 2. The nature of MIS now becomes clearer. Candida and virus are major factors; in the next chapter we will discuss what may be the most fascinating and surprising part of the picture—parasites.

REFERENCES

1. Dennis, D., Miller, M.J., Peterson, C.G. Candida septicemia. *Surg Gynecol Obstet.*, 1964; 119:520-530.
2. Gottlieb, M.S., Schroff, R., *et al.* Pneumocystis carinii pneumonia and mucosal candidiasis in previously healthy homosexual men. *New Eng J Med.*, 1981; 305:1425.
3. Bland, J. *Candida albicans: an unsuspecting problem.* Resource monograph, Dept. of Nutritional Biochemistry, University of Puget Sound, Washington, 1984.
4. Salvin, S.B. Endotoxin in pathogenic fungi. *J Immunol.*, 1952; 69:89-99.
5. Maibach, H.I., Kligman, A.M. The biology of experimental human cutaneous moniliasis (*Candida albicans*). *Arch Dermatol.*, 1962; 85:233-254.
6. Mourad, S., Friedman, L. Pathogenicity of Candida. *J Bacteriol.*, 1961; 81:550-556.
7. Martin, M.V., *et al.* An investigation of the role of true hyphae production in the pathogenesis of experimental oral candidosis. *Sab J Med Vet Mycology*, 1984; 22:471-76.
8. Rippon, J.W. Candidiasis and the pathogenic yeast. In: *Medical Mycology: The Pathogenic Fungi and the Pathogenic Actinomycetes*, W.B. Saunders, Philadelphia, 1982.
9. Louria, D.B., Brayton, R.G. A substance in blood lethal for *Candida albicans. Nature*, 1964; 201:309.
10. Nelson, R.D., Herron, M.J., *et al.* Two mechanisms of inhibition of human lymphocyte proliferation by soluble yeast mannan polysaccharide. *Infect Immunol.*, 1984; 43:1041-46.
11. Valdez, J.C., Meson, O.E., *et al.* Suppression of humoral response during the course of Candida albicans infection in mice. *Mycopathologia*, 1984; 88:61-63.
12. Schwab, J.H. Suppression of the immune response bymicroorganism. *Bacteriol Rev.*, 1975;39:121-43.
13. Stobo, J.D., *et al.* Suppressor derived lymphocytes in fungal infection. *J Clin Invest.*, 1976; 57:319-28.
14. Chilgren, R.A., Neuwissen, H.J. The cellular immune defect in Chronic mucocutaneous candidiasis. *Lancet*, 1969; i:1286-88.
15. Carlson, E. Enhancement by Candida albicans of Staphylococcus aureus, Serratia marcescens, and Streptococcus faecalis in the establishment of infection in mice. *Infection & Immunity*, 1983; 39(1):193.
16. Macmillan, B.G., Law, E.J., Holder, I.A. Experience with Candida infections in the burn patient. *Arch Surg.*, 1972; 104:509.
17. Truss, C.O. The role of Candida albicans in human illness. *J Orthomol Psychiatry*, 1981; 10:228-38.
18. Gentles, J.C., La Touche, C.J. Yeasts as human and animal pathogens. In: A.H. Rose and J.S. Harrison (eds.), *The Yeasts*, vol.1, London, Academic Press, 1969.
19. Sanchez, A., *et al.* Role of sugars in human neutrophilic phagocytosis. *Am J Clin Nutr.*, 1973; 26:180-187.
20. Bernstein, J., Alpert, S., Nauss, K.M., Suskind, R. Depression of lymphocyte transformation following oral glucose ingestion. (abstract) *Am J Clin Nutr.*, 1977; 30:613.
21. Burkitt, D.P. Relationships between diseases and their etiological significance. *Am J Clin Nutr.*, 1977; 30:262-67.

22. Kirsner, J.B., Shorter, R.G. Recent developments in "non-specific" inflamatory bowel disease. *New Eng J Med.*, 1982; 306:775.

23. Beisel, W.R. Malnutrition and the immune response. In: *Biochemistry of Nutrition*, Neuberger A., and Jukes, T.H. (eds.), University Park Press, Baltimore, 1979.

24. Caruso, L.J. Vaginal moniliasis after tetracycline therapy. *Am J Obstet Gynecol.*, 1964; 90:374.

25. Folb, P.I, Trounce, J.R. Immunological aspects of Candida infection complicating steroid and immunosuppressive drug therapy. *Lancet*, 1970; 2:1112.

26. Porter, P.S., Lyle, J.S. Yeast vulvovaginitis due to oral contraceptives. *Arch Dermatol Syphilogr.*, 1966; 93:402.

27. Kane, FJ Jr., Anderson, W.B. A fourth occurance of oral moniliasis during tranquilizer therapy. *Am J Psychiatry*, 1964; 120:1199.

28. Seelig, M.S. Mechanisms by which antibiotics increase the incidence and severity of candidiasis and alter the immunological defenses. *Bacteriological Rev.*, 1966; 30(2):442-459.

29. Rippon, J.W. *Medical Mycology*, Second Edition. WB Saunders Co. Philadelphia, 1982.

30. Odds, F.C. *Candida and Canidosis.* Baltimore, University Park Press, 1979, pp 82-85.

31. Cross, W.G. Oral reactions to penicillin. *Br Med J.*, 1949; 1:171.

32. Geiger, A.J., *et al.* Mycotic endocarditis and meningitis. *Yale J Biol & Med.*, 1946; 18:259.

33. Wessler S, Browne HR: Candida albicans (monilia albicans) infection with blood stream invasion; report of a case with a strain clinically resistant to sulfonamide drugs and to penicillin in vitro. *Ann Int Med.*, 1945; 22:886-89.

34. Campbell, C.C., Saslaw, S. Enhancement of growth of certain fungi by streptomycin. *Proc Soc Exp Biol Med.*, 1949; 70:562-68.

35. Seligmann, E. Virulence enhancing activities of Aureomycin on Candida albicans. *Proc Soc Exp Biol Med.*, 1952; 79:481-84.

36. Isenberg HD, Pisano M.A., Carito S.L., Berkman, J.I. Factors leading to overt monilial disease. I. Preliminary studies of the ecological relationship between Candida albicans and intestinal bacteria. *Antibiot Chemotherapy*, 1960; 10:353-63.

37. Ambrose, C.T., Coons, A.H. Studies on antibody production. *J Exp Med.*, 1963; 117:1075-88.

38. Munoz, J., Geister, R. Inhibition of phagocytosis by aureomycin. *Proc Soc Exp Biol Med.*, 1950; 75:367-370.

39. Keye, J.D. Jr., Magee, W.E. Fungal diseases in a general hospital. A study of 88 patients. *Am J Clin Pathol.*, 1956; 26:1235-53.,

40. Klein, J.J., Watanakunskorn, C. Hospital-acquired fungemia. Its natural course and clinical significance. *Am J Med.*, 1979; 67:51.

41. Barrett, B.W., Volwiler, W.M., Kirby, M.M., Jensen, C.R. Fatal systemic moniliasis following pancreatitis. *Arch Int Med.*, 1957; 99:209-13.

42. Lurie, M.B. The reticulo-endothelial system, cortisone, and thyroid function: their relation to native resistance to infection. *Ann N.Y. Acad Sci.*, 1961; 88:83-98.

43. Frenkel, J.K. Role of corticosteroids as predisposing factors in fungal diseases. *Lab Invest.*, 1962; 11:1192-1208.

44. Gorczyca, L.R., McCarty, R.T. Effects of prolonged low dosage antibiotic administration and superimposed Candida albicans infection on goat serum proteins. *Antibiot Chemother.*, 1959; 9:587-95.

45. Rosenberg, E.W., Belew, P.W., Skinner, R.B., Crutcher, N. Response to: Crohn's disease and psoriasis. *New Eng J Med.*, 1983; 308(2):101.

46. Horowitz, B.J., *et al.* Sugar chromatography studies in recurrent Candida vulvovaginitis. *J Reproductive Med.*, 1984; 29(7):441.

47. Diddle, A.W., Gardner, W.H., Williamson, P.J., O'Connor, K.A. Oral contraceptive medications and vulvovaginal candidiasis. *Obstet Gynecol.*, 1969; 34:373.

48. Wied, G.L., Davis, M.E., *et al.* Statistical evaluation of the effect of hormonal contraceptives on the cytologic smear pattern. *Obstet Gynecol.*, 1966; 27:327.

49. Miles, M.R., Olsen, L., Rogers, A. Recurrent vaginal candidiasis; importance of an intestinal reservoir. *JAMA*, 1977; 238:1836-37.

50. Witkin, S.S., Yu, I.R., Ledger, W.J. Inhibition of Candida albicans-induced lymphocyte proliferation by lymphocyte and sera from women with recurrent vaginitis. *Am J Obstet Gynecol.*, 1983; 147:809-11.

51. Goldman, H.J., *et al.* Monilial cystitis effective treatment with instillations of amphotericin B. *JAMA*, 1960; 174:359-62.

52. Keeney,E.L. Candida asthma. *Ann Int Med.*, 1951; 34: 223-227.

53. Pepys, J., *et al.* Candida albicans precipitins in respiratory disease in man. *J Allergy*. 1968; 41:305-310.

54. James, J., Warin, R.P. An assessment of the role of Candida albicans and food yeasts in chronic urticaria. *Br J Derm.*, 1971; 84: 227-237.

55. Editorial. Moniliasis in the urinary tract. *JAMA*, 1960; 174: 405-6.

56. Swartz, D.A., Harrington, P., Wilcox, R. Candidal epididymitis treated with ketoconazole. (letter) *New Eng J Med.*, 1988;319(22):1485.

57. Novick, R. Antibiotics: use in animal feed. *Science*, 1979; 204:908-11.

58. Anonymous. Antibiotics in milk. *Br Med J.*, 1963: 1491-92.

59. "Antibiotic Food Additives: The Prospect of Doing Without" Farmline, U.S. Dept of Agriculture. Dec. 1980.

60. Harris, N.V., Weiss, N.S., and Nolan, C.M., The role of poultry and meats in the etiology of campylobacter jejuni/coli enteritis. *Am J Public Health*, 1986; 76: 407-11.

61. Waisman, M. Genital moniliasis as a conjugal infection. *Arch Dermat Syph.*, 1954: 70: 718.

62. Goldberg, P.K., Kozinn, P.J., *et al.* Incidence and significance of candiduria. *JAMA*, 1979; 241: 582.

63. Powell, N.B., Powell, E.B., *et al.* Allergy of the lower urinary tract. *J Urol.*, 1972; 107: 631.

64. Walter, C. Allergy as a cause of genitourinary symptoms: Clinical considerations. *Ann Allergy*, 1958; 10:158.

CHAPTER 5

PARASITES

We were informed by one medical investigator that 80% of patients might be infected with parasites. This news was stunning in its implications.

Since our sojourns in medical school, we agreed that the idea of parasitic infestation always brought to mind the picture of rain forests and tropical rivers in the Orient, the Amazon or the Congo. For years we thought that it did not concern our patients here in the temperate climate of hygienic U.S.A. We never bothered to learn more than the bare essentials about diagnosis and treatment of these complex creatures. Several years ago, things began to change. Dr. Warren Levin from New York told us about a Dr. Louis Parrish, a psychiatrist who was doing anoscopy (examination of the anus with a scope) on many of his patients and taking direct rectal swabs for *Entameba histolytica* (E. *histolyica*) and *Giardia lamblia* (G. *lamblia*). After we contacted Dr. Parrish directly, he informed us that he was getting about 80% positive indications for the presence of parasitic infections with his method! This news was stunning. Though at first we were skeptical, we have since ventured through many more stages of discovery and found that parasites are indeed an important part of illness in the U.S.A. Interestingly, for years both naturopathic physicians and colonic therapists have claimed that many of their patients have parasitic infection(s).

Little by little, by using available medical techniques for examining stool samples for parasites, we began to uncover numerous, previously unsuspected, parasitic infections. Then by going a step beyond routine stool examination techniques, we found much larger numbers of parasite cases. We simply combined standard stool examination with stool purges. The purge is a laxative which flushes out parasites.

Although any organism that invades and feeds upon another organism can be defined as parasitic, there is a class of medical organism specifically called parasites. These organisms are not bacteria, viruses, or fungi (all of which are "parasitic").

Medical parasites fall into three categories:

1. Worms (roundworms, flatworms, and flukes)
2. Arthropods (little insects like ticks and mites)
3. Protozoal (single cell) organisms like *Entameba histolytica* (E. *histolytica*) or *Giardia lamblia* (G. *lamblia*)

Parasites, we now understand, may be a major contributing factor to CFS. As far as CFS is concerned, we will discuss, primarily, *Giardia lamblia, Entameba histolytica,* and *Ascaris lumbricoides* (A. *lumbricois*.). There are several others which we will touch upon, but for our purpose, these we have learned, are the most important.

The class of disease-causing organisms called parasites includes hundreds of species ranging from microscopic one cell protozoa to tapeworms, some of which measure three feet in length! Parasites can be introduced into our body through contamination of food and water, or exposure to wind, soil, insects, animals, birds and fish. Pets carry parasites, many of which can infect humans. Pets can also carry fleas, ticks, and other arthropods which in turn can carry smaller infectious organisms like *Borrelia*, a coiled spirochete shaped parasite that causes Lyme disease, and *Yersinia pestis*, which causes the dreaded bubonic plague. This is an amazing microcosm of disease, not all of which pertains to CFS.

The parasites have been coevolving with man for millions of years, and like viruses and fungi, their presence in the body serves no known purpose. Indeed, infection with parasites taxes and suppresses immune function and may lead to serious illness and even death.[1]

We have learned, for example, that a type of cancer called Burkitt's lymphoma often develops from the interaction of Epstein-Barr virus and chronic malaria infection. Since malaria is a parasitic disease, it is reasonable that other parasite/virus or other microbe connections may play a role in human disease. It is not really a long shot, even in spanking clean USA, to observe that many people with mysterious disease show evidence of parasites, often along with yeast or virus or bacteria.

Even though there is more parasitic disease in the tropics, there has always been parasite infection in our temperate climes.[2] Furthermore, a number of 20th century factors have resulted in increased risk:

1. Widespread travel:

   More Americans are traveling to parts of the world where the water, food, and soil may be contaminated with parasites. Many not only are infected themselves, but may carry the organism back home where infection of family members is possible (though not likely).

   In addition, thousands of soldiers returning from Southeast Asia in the period from 1963 to 1975 were harboring a variety of parasites, including chronic and potentially lethal infections of the intestine, lungs, liver and central nervous system.[3]

2. Modern international food distribution:

   Today, food is flown to the U.S. from every corner of the globe. Testing for parasites is virtually impossible as they are usually carried as eggs or cysts, not visible organisms. Proper handling and cooking, of course, reduces risk of infection, but problems still arise.

3. Popularity of new ethnic foods:

   Any meat, fish or fowl which is not thoroughly cooked can carry parasites, but ethnic dishes containing semi-cooked meat may be safe if properly marinated or smoked.[4-6]

4. The sexual revolution:

   Individuals who have numerous sexual partners increase their risk for trichomoniasis, a venereal parasite that affects mainly women. Contrary to popular belief, however, men are often infected, and may be asymptomatic carriers for many years. In addition, the organism can cause chronic urethritis and prostatitis, and may account for up to 20% of non-gonorrheal venereal disease in men.[7] It is likely that unusual practices such as oral-anal sex could lead to contagion of parasitic disease, since most parasitic diseases are spread through fecal contamination.

5. Influx of immigration and travel from tropical and subtropical regions:

   Parasitic infections predominate in tropical and subtropical regions of the world. Although this is certainly no cause for alarm or xenophobia, the incidence of parasitic infections in immigrants from Asia, the South Pacific, Haiti, Mexico, Central and South America far exceeds that found in the general population.[8-10]

Dr. Lucrece Dowell, of Dowell Laboratory in Phoenix, Arizona, theorizes that much of the parasite infection in the USA comes from produce grown in irrigated fields. Dr. Dowell observes that the workers in these fields may use the irrigation ditches as latrines. The untreated water then gets sprayed on the growing produce. If these fruits and vegetables are not well washed before consumption, we can get exposed to parasite eggs. If normal defenses in the stomach and intestines are not adequate, we could get parasitic infection. You might experience this infection as a mild "flu." This mild "flu" might not get better. It could linger for years and could trigger the CFS.

THE PLAIN TRUTH ABOUT PARASTITES

Myth: Parasite infections are rare.

Reality: Based on medical records and disease patterns, health experts claim that three out of every five Americans (60%) will experience parasitic infections in their lifetime.[11] We can understand this better by looking at a few common examples.

Public health experts report that roughly 25% of the world's population, including over 1 million Americans are infected with *Ascaris lumbricoides* (A. *lumbricoides*) also known as roundworms. They spend part of their life cycle in the soil.[12] Infection by this organism can therefore occur by eating contaminated food or the introduction of microscopic ascaris eggs into the mouth by the hands after contact with contaminated soil. In dry, windy areas, infection may even take place by inhalation of microscopic airborne eggs.

At this moment, 20 to 30 million Americans are infected with the nematode *Enterobiusvermicularis* (E. *vermicularis*) also known as pinworms.[13] Once again contamination is rapid, and a short time after one individual becomes infected, every member of the family or communal group member may become exposed. Only prompt treatment can prevent its spread.

The protozoa, *Toxoplasma gondii* (T. *gondii*), causes another parasitic disease called toxoplasmosis, which reportedly infects up to half of the world's population! Typically T. *gondii* inhabits the blood and lymphatic fluids. In one large study, American army recruits were tested for antibodies to this organism. Twenty percent of men from the east coast, three percent from the Rocky Mountain states, and eight percent from the west coast were found to be infected; overall, fourteen percent of recruits tested positive for the organism.[14] Could this be a factor in CFS?

Health experts now believe that toxoplasmosis may establish a chronic infective state in humans much like EBV, controlled by a healthy immune system, but ready to proliferate if the body's immune defenses are impaired. There is support for this theory in the rapidly increasing incidence of serious toxoplasmosis in AIDS patients and in other immune suppressed individuals.[15]

Trichomoniasis is the sexually transmitted parasite which can be chronic in both sexes. Public health experts have estimated that up to 25% of sexually active Americans may be infected.[16] This is another possible spoke in the ever enlarging wheel that may comprise CFS.

Overall, however, amebiasis and giardiasis may be the two most important parasites involved with CFS. Diseases associated with ameba are well known. Humans harbor a number of amebic strains, only one of which seems to cause serious illness. Surveys show that infection with this strain, *Entameba histolytica*, may be as high as 5% of the entire U.S. population (over 10 million people). In some areas with poor sanitation, however, rates as high as 50% have been reported.[17] World-wide, there are an estimated one billion people infested with this parasite.

Giardia lamblia, the intestinal parasite, infects another 8 to 10 million Americans.[18] Giardia is a common cause of traveler's diarrhea, but gastrointestinal symptoms can persist for many months or years. Unfortunately, even when symptoms abate, the organism may still actively proliferate in the intestine, and this intermittent characteristic may lull both victim and doctor into neglect or mis-diagnosis.

One need not travel outside the U.S. to become exposed to giardia. A number of wild animals serve as host to the organism, and appear to be responsible for the frequent contamination of ponds and mountain streams.[19] Giardiasis is one of the most common waterborne diseases in the U.S., and has been responsible for repeated outbreaks affecting thousands of people.[20,21] It is responsible for many of the illnesses experienced by people when fishing, hiking, or participating in other wilderness activities.

Children are certainly susceptible. Before children develop an awareness of proper hygiene, they may pick up giardia at day care centers and schools. This is worrisome because they are also less able to articulate the intestinal distress from their ensuing infection. Many health experts consider giardia to be one of the most dangerous intestinal parasites because it typically infects the duodenal segment of the small intestine. Since this is the area where over 90% of nutrient absorption takes place, chronic giardiasis can be a major cause of undernutrition or malnutrition.[22] Injury due to giardia of the intestinal wall is also common, and evidence suggests that this may lead to subsequent reactivation of the latent Epstein-Barr virus.[23]

One patient whom we puzzled over suffered severe pain in the right upper quadrant of her abdomen. She had severe digestive disturbances, dizziness, nausea, and of course the intense fatigue characteristic of CFS. We discovered giardia in her stool and her Upper G.I. X-Rays showed her to have duodenitis, or inflammation of the duodenum. This is a common condition which is sometimes considered to be a sign of early peptic ulcer disease. When we told the radiologist about the giardia, he looked it up in his reference books and discovered that this common duodenitis was also characteristic of giardia. He was surprised. How many radiologists around the country do you suppose would be surprised by this knowledge?

Blastocystis hominis (B. *hominis*) is a mysterious and controversial protozoal parasite—or pathogenic fungal/yeast form—depending on which expert you consult. Evidence is continually accumulating which supports the pathogenic role of this organism. It has been implicated in outbreaks of diarrhea in families. It is fairly often present in CFS patients. Recent work indicates that it respond to treatment with medications such as Metronidazole. We feel it could contribute to CFS.

Cryptosporidium is a fairly obscure protozoa which is the cause of acute diarrhea epidemics when civic water supplies are contaminated. It resists sterilization by chlorinated water. There is no drug on the U.S. market which treats Cryptosporidium. This is not considered to be a problem because the acute cases are considered to be "self-limited," and the chronic cases are considered to be "non-pathogenic." If that were true, it would mean that we will never need a treatment for this elusive little parastite. The authors of this book treat cryptosporidium with herbs (chapter 10).

There are textbooks filled with exotic names of parasites—*Endolimax nana*, *Entameba coli*, hookworms, flukes, pins, tapes, malaria, etc., etc. These supposedly uncommon pathogens can wreak havoc when they are not diagnosed. They often present problems even when we diagnose them. Although they do not seem to have statistical significance in the CFS picture (in the USA), they do occur but rarely contribute to CFS.

Myth: It is easy to tell if you have parasites because there are obvious signs.

Reality: Most individuals, even many doctors, overlook this problem because parasites often do not cause the classic symptoms of gastrointestinal distress. In actuality, many parasites do not produce significant diarrhea at all, and those that do may only cause such symptoms at one stage of their life cycle. It can be very sneaky.

Myth: Almost all parasite infections are cleared up after the organism completes one life cycle.

Reality: Many parasites can establish long term infection states by evading or suppressing immune system control. This leads to autoinocculaton (self infection). In one recent study of chronic giardiasis, the mean duration of infection was found to be 3.3 years,[24] and infection with *Strongyloides*, an intestinal worm, often persists for 20 or 30 years.[25] There are estimates that many parasites can survive for decades in humans.

Myth: Detection of parasite infection is easy.

Reality: This may be the most harmful myth, since most parasite infections are probaby missed by standard testing procedures. Spot stool analysis is still the most commonly prescribed test for parasites even though it has been found to be inadequate in most cases.[26] At the very least, such tests should be conducted three to four times, 5 to 7 days apart, in order to evaluate the presence of parasites. Even then, there are significant problems with this method of testing. As we mentioned, many parasites spend much of their life cycle outside the intestine, and no number of stool tests will detect them. *Ascaris* worms, for example, have a pulmonary phase where the parasite larvae reside in the lungs and later migrate through the bronchial tubes. During this time, as well as in the first 2 to 3 months in the intestinal stage, the organism produces no eggs, and will not show up in stool tests. [27]

As will be described in Chapter 10 and the appendix, the mixed infection syndrome approach to parasite evaluation includes a more sensitive and accurate method of stool testing, and sometimes specific blood tests and careful attention to other elements in standard blood tests which may alert us to parasites.

PERSPECTIVE

It is not our intention to paint a bleak picture of overwhelming peril from parasitic infection. The diagnosis and treatment of parasites is perhaps the most satisfying of all infectious agents which physicians may encounter The diagnosis is often iron clad, which is more than we can ever say for pure CFS. The medications and even the herbs which we use for parasites are highly effective. Even when the parasites are not diagnosed and treated, they may resolve through boosting our own immune system function. However, when other factors impair our defenses, it could take months, years or decades to eliminate the parasite, and during that time, the parasite adds significantly to the toxic burden on the body's immune system. As such, these organisms play an important and increasingly common role in the CFS. Parasites produce endotoxins as do other microbial organisms such as yeast and bacteria. In addition, parasitic damage to intestinal membranes is often severe, allowing for increased absorption of these endotoxins and other damaging material through the bowel wall and into the bloodstream.[28]

A major interactive cycle exists, in fact, between parasites and allergy, and researchers are beginning to see marked similarities in the body's reaction to both disorders.[29]

One well known immune response to parasites is the production of specialized combat white cells called eosinophils. These cells contain a number of highly toxic proteins and oxygen radicals with which they fight micropathogens. In addition, they release biochemicals called leukotrienes and prostaglandins which initiate inflammation in the surrounding tissue. This "alarm" mechanism is useful for attracting other immune cells into the fray, but chronic infection can cause eosinophil levels to increase to the point where they themselves damage tissue, resulting in pain and inflammation.

The body's major response to allergy, on the other hand, is distinguished by an increase in antibodies, primarily immunoglobulin E (IgE). Once again, the allergic reaction triggers a chain reaction involving inflammation and other immune cells. Recent work sheds light on allergic reactions, perhaps from parasite infections, stimulating the production of eosinophils.[30] Note that parasites, like allergy, stimulate the production of IgE.[31]

Important similarities and interactions exist between parasites and Candida infection. Entry of parasites into the body, for example, is most often by the oral route, and stomach acid is the first major defense. The highly acidic hydrochloric acid (HCL) in our stomach is crucial to our defense against destroying pathogenic microbes. There are very few pathogenic micoorganisms which can survive the highly acid environment of the stomach. Candida over-growth, however, can damage the HCL producing cells,[32] and may therefore increase the risk for parasite infection.[33] This is one reason we chose to discuss candidiasis before parasites in this book. In its fungal phase, the Candida organism sends root-like structures into the lining of the intestine. Numerous parasites can also penetrate this lining to a similar degree by imbedding themselves in surface tissue. *Entameba histolytica*, in fact, produces an enzyme which literally digests the intestinal lining, creating "foxholes." This clever little invader then lives and reproduces in the resulting pocket. In such cases, the invasive combination of fungus and parasite ultimately leads to immune suppression.[34] It is also easy to see how these organisms may initiate a cycle of malabsorption and nutrient deficiency leading to malnutrition, which further lowers an individual's defense against all pathogens associated with CFS.[35]

With all this background in parasitology, we can now begin to see how it may apply to CFS. To us, the important aspect of all this is really our personal experience in diagnosing and treating various parasitic infections. In our experience, between 30% and 40% of patients with CFS have detectable parasites. Easily one half of those will get obvious and swift improvement from treatment (Chapter 10 and appendix.) This in itself is a significant figure. Since CFS patients often shuttle from doctor to doctor seeking help, we often see patients with undiagnosed parasitic infections who have tried numerous unsuccessful treatments.

When a patient who has been to 5 or 10 doctors without help has parasites detected, that patient has about a 50% chance of swift improvement. We have seen this kind of response repeatedly. When many such patients respond so dramatically, it gives further support to our contention that parasites are a major contributor of the CFS puzzle.

Case History

J.S. was a 45 year old businessman who had been severely depressed for two years when he came to see us. Despite having seen three physicians, his depression progressed to the point of his considering suicide. He suffered low grade fevers and sweats. He was clearly unable to work, and his once prosperous retail business was failing. He was virtually bedridden. He had been treated, unsuccessfully, with anti-depressant medication, prescribed to him by a physician with an exceptional reputation in his field.

None of J.S.'s physicians thought it pertinent that the patient began feeling ill shortly after a business trip to the Orient. During that trip he contracted a *severe* case of traveler's diarrhea. The diarrhea resolved itself in about a week, but the patient continued to feel fatigued and depressed. These feelings became progressively worse until he sought medical care. We might add that prior to developing traveler's diarrhea, he had been perfectly healthy.

When we saw J.S. after two years of his on-going odyssey, his history was striking. It just seemed like sound medicine for us to check J.S. for parasites after his diarrheal history. In our opinion, it should be standard medicine to evaluate for evidence of parasitic infection whenever this type of case history is given.

We did a thorough work up on J.S., including physical examination, various chemistries, antibody tests, and a stool purge (laxative) for parasites and yeast. The purge test, which we often recommend to detect stool parasites, has been highly effective. In this case it diagnosed J.S. to be infested with *Dientameba histolytica*— amebiasis. Ameba are tiny parasites, not much bigger than a white blood cell. And as we said earlier, there are almost one billion people in the world who are infested with amebiasis, obviously not a rare infection. What is not obvious is how many people develop fatigue due to it. We see many people who tolerate it fairly well. But we are all individuals with individual responses to infections like ameba. J.S.'s response to amebiasis was depression and fatigue. We began J. S. on a course of Metronidazole and Iodoquinol, two medical drugs commonly prescribed for this infection. We also put J. S. on a program of improved diet with selected vitamin and mineral supplementation, which are not standard for most doctors but are almost universally used in our approach.

In ten days, he was completely cured!

His depression was gone; he resumed his life at full speed. His "CFS" was gone.

What lessons can we learn from this case? First, let us assume that the obvious is true. Let us say that the patient contracted amebiasis which was not discovered for two years. Let us also say that the persistent amebiasis caused the CFS and depression. It follows then, that the treatment of this parasitic infection worked and resolved this patient's depression and fatigue almost instantly. In the context of CFS, this case could teach us many lessons. The most important of these may be that "CFS" can often be an ordinary disease which is difficult to diagnose. This was not a mixed infectious syndrome because it was evidently a single infection. The case brings up the tantalizing question of how many supposed CFS patients are readily curable by proper diagnosis. One thing which this case definitely does not do is give us any significant clue as to the ultimate cause or cure of *true* CFS, if such a thing exists.

The most important pragmatic lesson for us is the idea that we must diagnose and treat the patient for whatever fatigue-causing condition he may be experiencing. Parasites are among the most common of treatable conditions associated with "CFS." The parasites which we see most frequently are G. *lamblia* and E. *histolytica*. These parasites were the cause of the J.S.'s amebiasis. A slightly distant third would be A. *lumbricoides*. These parasites are common and highly treatable, both with medical and herbal approaches.

The conclusion which we make is that certain parasites are a significant part of the mixed infectious nature of CFS. We feel that parasites are perhaps the most standard element which standard medical practice overlooks. Parasites are highly diagnosable and treatable by orthodox methodology. They require, however, the very best of orthodoxy. The doctor must have a clear index of suspicion, must order and conduct the proper tests, properly interpret them and, of course, order appropriate treatment. If all this were done on all patients labeled with "CFS," perhaps 20% of such patients would be promptly cured of their affliction. That is why parasites are vital in the CFS picture.

Let us now look at the last and seemingly least important of the four horsemen of CFS: bacteria.

REFERENCES

1. Crewe, W., Haddock, D.R.W. *Parasites and Human Disease*, New York, Wiley Medical Publications, 1985.
2. *Parasites and Western Man*, R.J. Donaldson (ed.), Baltimore, University Park Press, 1979.
3. Hakim, S.Z., Genta, R.M. Fatal disseminated strongyloidiasis in a Vietnam War veteran. *ARCH Pathol Lab Med.*, 1986; 110(9):809.
4. Modern international food distribution.
5. Adams, K.O., Jungkind, D.L., Bergquist, E.J., Wirts, C.W. Intestinal fluke infection as a result of eating sushi. *Am J Clin Pathol.*, 1986; 86(5):688.
6. Ishizuka, T., Ishizuka, A. A case of diphyllobothriasis due to eating masou-sushi. *Med J Aust.*, 1986; 145(2):114.
7. Goldman, D.R. Hold the sushi [letter]. *JAMA*, 1985; 253(17):2495.
8. Parish, R.A. Intestinal Parasites in Southeast Asian refugee children. *West J Med.*, 1985; 143(1):47.
9. Langley, A.J., Baker, C.C. Health screening of immigrants. *Med J Aust.*, 1987; 146(8):449.
10. Proceedings of the Sixth International Congress of Parasitology. 24-29 August 1986. *Int J Parasitol.*, 1987; 17(2):301.
11. *Parasitic Diseases*, J.M. Mansfield (ed.) New York, Marcel Dekker, 1981.
12. Plorde, J.J. Intestinal nematodes. In: *Harrison's Principles of Internal Medicine*. G.W. Thorne, *et al.* (Eds.) New York, McGraw-Hill, 1977.
13. Basch, P.F. Enterobiasis. In: *Public Health and Preventive Medicine*, 11th edition, J.M. Last, (ed.) New York, Appleton-Century-Crofts, 1980.
14. Feldman, H.A. Toxoplasmosis: an overview. *Bull New York Acad Med.*, 1974; 50:110.

15. Rotterdam, H. Tissue diagnosis of selected AIDS-related opportunistic infections. *Am J Surg Pathol.*, 1987; 11 (Suppl 1):3.
16. Jirovec, O., Petru, M. Trichomonas vaginalis and trichomonas. In: *Advances in Clinical Pathology*, vol 6, B Dawes (ed.) London, Academic Press, 1968.
17. Elsdon-Dew, R. The epidemiology of amebiasis. *Adv Parasitol.*, 1968; 6:1.
18. Ash, L.R., Orihel, T.C. *Atlas of Human Parasitology*, 2nd edition. Chicago, American Society of Clinical Pathologists Press, 1984.
19. Brady, P.G., Wolfe, J.C. Waterborne giardiasis. *Ann Int Med.*, 1974; 81:498.
20. Moore, G.T., Cross, W.M., *et al.* Epidemic giardiasis at a ski resort. *New Eng J Med.*, 1969: 281:402.
21. Shaw, P.K., Brodsky, R.E., *et al.* A communitywide outbreak of giardiasis with evidence of transmission by a municipal water supply. *Ann Int Med.*, 1977; 87:426.
22. Hoskins, L.C., *et al.* Clinical giardiasis and intestinal malabsorption. *Gastroenterology*, 1967; 53:265.
23. DuBois, R.E., Seeley, J.K., *et al.* Chronic mononucleosis syndrome. *S Med J.*, 1984; 77(11):1376.
24. Chester, A.C., MacMurray, F.G., Restifo, M.D., Mann, O. Giardiasis as a chronic disease. *Dig Dis Sci.*, 1985; 30(3):215.
25. Plorde, J.J. Intestinal nematodes. In: *Harrison's Principles of Internal Medicine*, 8th edition. G.W. Thorne, R.D. Adams, *et al.*, (eds.) New York, McGraw-Hill, 1977.
26. Guerrant, R.L., Shields, D.S., *et al.* Evaluation and diagnosis of acute infectious diarrhea. *Am J Med.*, 1985; 78(68):91.
27. Brown, H-W. *Basic Clinical Parasitology*, 4th edition. New York, Appleton-Century-Crofts, 1975.
28. Mackenzie, C.D., Gatrill, A.J., *et al.* Inflamatory response to parasites. *Parasitology*, 1987; 94 Suppl:9.
29. Ferguson, A., Miller, H.R.P. Role of the mast cell in the defense against gut parasite. In: *The Mast Cell.* J. Pepys, A.M. Edwards, (eds.) Tunbridge Wells, Eng., Pitman Medical Publishing, 1979
30. Venge, P., Hakansson, L., Peterson, C.G.B. Eosinophil activation in allergic disease. *Arch Allergy Appl Immun.*, 1987; 82:333.
31. Lynch, N.R., *et al.* IgE antibody against surface antigens of Leishmania promastigotes in American cutaneous leishmaniasis. *Parasite Immunol.*, 1986; 8(2)109.
32. Holmstrom, B., Wallensten, S., Frisk, A. Presence of fungi in gastric and duodenal ulcers. *Acta Chir Scand.*, 1959; 117:215.
33. Plorde, J.J. Minor protozoan diseases. In: *Harrison's Principles of Internal Medicine*, 8th edition, G.W. Thorne, R.D. Adams, *et al.* (eds.) New York, McGraw Hill, 1977.
34. Schwab, J.H. Suppression of the immune response by microorganism. *Bacteriol Rev.*, 1975; 39:121.
35. Chandra, R.K. Nutrition, immunity, and infection: present knowledge and future directions. *Lancet*, 1983; 1(8326):688.

CHAPTER 6

BACTERIA

Some causes of chronic fatigue are found in a sea of obscure bacterial infections.

We said in the previous chapter that bacterial infections are seemingly less important in contributing to CFS. Our opinion may change in time. Recent research has begun to reveal that many bacterial infections may be important in CFS but are undiagnosable using today's clinical methods. How might hidden bacterial infections help us understand CFS?

Remember NSU and NGU? NSU referred to a non-specific urethritis, while NGU referred to the non-gonococcal urethritis (or non-bacterial urethritis). These were medical descriptions for mysterious inflammations of the urethra which sometimes followed venereal exposure. For men it was less affectionately called "the strain" owing to the pain and mucus discharge they experienced at the end of the penis. Women suffered with urinary "burning" and a vaginal discharge. It took years before laboratory advances revealed this condition was due to a micropathogenic organism called *Chlamydia*.

Today chlamydia is considered the most common infection of all sexually transmitted infections, (although it is not always venereal), and possibly responsible for about one half of all infertility problems in women. Chlamydia has been difficult to diagnose because it is difficult to culture. The organism has no cell wall and does not grow in the culture material used to test for most bacteria. Before accurate tests became available, chlamydial infections were often treated empirically (meaning trial and error—or better yet—trial and success); the burning sensation on urination or intercourse and the slight mucoid discharge from the urethra or the vagina responded to antibiotics, even though no organism could be found. Even though chlamydia was a less dramatic infection than gonorrhea or syphilis, the condition required a lengthier period of antibiotic therapy—three weeks versus only five to ten days. However, before doctors learned how to identify and treat chlamydia correctly, it was often only partially treated. The partially treated infection may then smolder indefintely, which may explain why chlamydia is an important bacterial contributor to the CFS in some patients.

What is the relationship of such hidden bacterial infections to CFS?

There was a professor in our medical school training, back in 1965, who stated that medicine had "conquered infectious disease." That statement should have reminded us of the government bureaucrat who urged the closing of all patent offices in 1900, because everything of importance had already been invented! Certainly we have made great advances in dealing with most infections, especially those that are bacterial. We have not, however, by any standard, conquered *all* infectious diseases. The prevalence of CFS attests to that unfortunate reality.

Many common bacterial infections such as strep throat, tonsillitis, sinusitis, bronchitis, cystitis, and perhaps that most insidious of all, acne, are serious contributors to CFS, with acne being the most common. It is remarkable how many CFS patients have provided us a history of extended treatment with antibiotics for their acne. This history was often followed by the development of mononucleosis or another systemic illness, which in some cases evolved into CFS. For some patients, this history dates back several decades! Every day we see new patients whose chronic health problems started after antibiotic treatment of some bacterial infection.

Let us describe an example, focusing on chlamydia, a genito-urinary tract infection, easily transmitted, difficult to isolate, stubborn and resistant to treatment. In daily medical practice, a doctor might treat such an infection without even testing for it. Such empirical treatment can be practical for the busy doctor and result in resolving the infection. It may start with a phone call from the patient complaining of urninary burning. Suppose we treat a case of apparent chlamydia empirically with antibiotics until it resolves. However, in some cases, after only two or three days symptoms may recur and the situation gets worse. This may occur even while the patient is still on antibiotics. Alternatively, suppose we have made a definitive diagnosis of chlamydia by using the fluorescent antibody technique. This is a highly reliable test when positive. (When negative it does not prove much.) Suppose the same thing happens: early improvement with treatment, followed by recurrence of the same or similar symptoms. Again, this is while the patient is still on the original antibiotic.

What has happened? Whether or not the chlamydia was proven, we now face several possibilities:

1. Something was wrong with the antibiotic—either the wrong dose, wrong type of antibiotic, or too low a potency in the batch (rare but possible).
2. a. Nothing was wrong with the antibiotic, but it killed too many friendly bacteria, creating a superinfection such as the Candida yeast.
   b. Parasites, especially vaginal trichomonas, might also flourish under such a circumstance.
   c. Herpes virus may also flare under this opportunity.
   d. It is also, of course, possible to develop a secondary bacterial infection in this ecology. Bacteria are sometimes the worst case, because the lethal and resistant bacteria prosper in these situations, *Clostridia, Staphlococcus, Gardnerella,* being some examples of the opportunistic forms typical in such situations.

When we look at the whole person and the seemingly infinite number of infections that are possible, we might lose the trees for the forest. Some of the problem with CFS are the overwhelming numbers of possibilities when we start to recognize that some obscure infection is causing the condition. In CFS it is important to find the specific bacterial "tree" and treat that infection. We need to ease the burden on the immune system. Every infection which we eradicate gives us more strength to defend ourselves, if we do not create a super-infection. Avoidance of that problem is addressed in our last two chapters.

Listed below are some of the unrecognized bacterial infections which can contribute to the development and existence of CFS:

1. A chronic gum infection often called *periodontitis,* which is a bacterial, *cellulitis* or tissue infection of the gums, which, when advanced, can erode the alveolar bone around the teeth.
2. *Lyme disease* caused by a sneaky twisty, corkscrew, bacterium called *Borrelia,* similar to syphilis yet not venereal in nature. A tick bite is the primary mode of transmission of this bacterium.
3. *Peptic ulcer* appears to be an infectious disease. Ulcer disease now appears to be caused by *Helicobacter pylori* (formerly *Campylobactor pylori*). What if the stress associated

with ulcer disease is caused by the ulcer and not the cause of it? There is some evidence now that H. *pylori* may be spread by drinking contaminated water. It's too soon to be sure, but some suggest that this problem may yet be another bacterial contributor of CFS.

4. *Acne,* owing to chronic bacterial infection of oil-secreting-glands of the skin. We do not doubt that this is an important player in CFS.
5. *Interstitial cystitis,* chronic bacteria or obscure or *mixed* infection of the deeper cells of the lining of the urinary bladder. Many women suffer from this condition leading to treatments involving antibiotics, unfortunately resulting in many cases of candidiasis.
6. *Chronic prostatitis,* which is often an incurable infection of the prostate gland. (Same possiblity as interstitial cystitis.)
7. *Chronic sinusitis,* a stubborn, sometimes incurable infection of the facial sinuses. (Same as chronic prostatitis.)

These are some of the many infections, the treatment of which is often frustrating and may lead to candidiasis and perhaps then to the Mixed Infection Syndrome (MIS) charateristic of so many cases of CFS. The medical problem in approaching these infections stems from the tunnel vision of standard medicine. The typical medical approach is to use an antibiotic if the infection seems evident. If the antibiotic fails, try another, then another, until either the patient or the doctor is exhausted or some toxic reaction forces termination of antibiotic therapy. In the chapter on treatment (10) we will discuss how to approach such problems using a combined therapy of strengthening the immune system while suppressing the bacterial organisms that have invaded.

We know that these infections can have surprising effects. The late Thomas McPherson Brown, M.D., the prominent rheumatologist from Georgetown University Medical School, roused medical controversy for decades by treating rheumatoid arthritis with ordinary antibiotics such as tetracycline. He felt that rheumatoid arthritis was often caused by chlamydia. He eventually published a number of papers showing good long term results. If he hadn't, why would he continue using this approach for decades? Dr. Brown's studies indicated that as many as 60% of rheumatoid arthritis patients improved with long term antibiotics.

We have had experiences that confirm Dr. Brown's work. We treated a lady with severe arthritis, fatigue, and chronic, refractory exudative tonsillitis. When all else failed, and as a last resort, she finally had a tonsillectomy. We were delightfully shocked to see her arthritis disappear *the next day after surgery*. More germane to this discussion, her CFS quickly resolved.

We have seen many such "coincidences" in our medical odyssey on the seas of obscure infection. If there is a chronic, deep rooted, antibiotic resistant, process of micro-abcesses in the tonsils, the above problems could logically result. Arthritis is often caused by infection. Fatigue is often caused by infection. If you remove the infection surgically, prompt improvement is a typical result. The same thing can be done with antibiotics, although it takes longer. We chose this example because of the dramatic and obvious response of CFS to removal of infection surgically.

Though candidiasis and EBV may be the whistle blowers, the culprit may be the bacterial infection. It is tragic when a highly treatable bacterial infection goes undiagnosed. It is almost as bad when the infection is known but tolerated because the antibiotics do not work. In the treatment chapter we will describe some combined approaches which have been successful with these stubborn infections.

We still need a philosophy and a plan to deal with the overall problem. Some day we may have a magic wand like "Bones," the doctor in the TV series Star Trek. He can wave an electronic probe over the body and get a reading on the patient's biochemical needs. Since we have not achieved that exalted level of technology, we must settle for our brains and our primitive testing. We can conjecture sufficiently to deduce reasonable strategy. Then we determine the tactics and go for it.

A rational approach to such a problem might be as follows.

a. We must be alert for many possibilities of bacterial infection, as well as the other classes of infection. We must do the appropriate laboratory studies to determine if any of the most likely suspicious organisms can be isolated. There are several satisfactory tests now available for detecting chlamydia. Their reliability approaches 90%, but that leaves at least 10% that are misleadingly false. Do not fall into the trap of blindly believing the lab studies, if they do not fit the apparent clinical picture. On the other hand, be ready to do any and all tests that may unravel the mystery. Lyme disease, for example, may lead to CFS. Once diagnosed, it will of course cease to be CFS and will be Lyme disease, but the fatigue is the same until you make the diagnosis. Any of the above infections can be the cause of chronic fatigue. Often all the tests will be negative.

Therefore:

b. Be willing to *treat empirically* the most likely organisms that seem to be causing CFS. Sometimes a therapeutic trial is the only way to make a tentative diagnosis. If the clinical picture is one of chronic fatigue, and candida and parasites have been eliminated as issues, the next action may best be a therapeutic trial of likely bacterial infections, perhaps including chlamydia. This fairly desperate course may make sense in such a case. Hippocrates said that *desperate conditions require desperate remedies.* Therapeutic trials in such a case can be done with some impunity since the therapies are usually much less toxic than the alternative of doing nothing. Therapy for bacteria can be relatively benign if we use precautionary *Lactobacillus acidophilus* and other beneficial forms of *Lactobacilli* (See treatment chapter).

It is increasingly apparent that we must become masters of medical deductive reasoning. It is glaringly obvious that the major weakness in the standard medical approach to CFS is its unwillingness to use deductive methods. If there is no clear technology for dealing with a problem, some contend it is best simply to abstain from doing anything. Those who believe this will fall back on the old standby phrase: "We've done all we can. You've got to learn to live with it." In our opinion, that's not good enough!

CHAPTER 7

OTHER CAUSES OF CHRONIC FATIGUE

Low grade chronic toxicity to lead, cadmium or mercury, must be considered in the differential diagnosis of chronic fatigue.

THE DIFFERENTIAL DIAGNOSIS

In medicine, there is the phrase, "differential diagnosis." When patients present themselves to a doctor, the doctor takes the presenting complaint and considers the most likely diagnosis, along with other possible diagnoses. The list of other possibilities is called the differential diagnosis. A sore throat, for example, might be the presenting symptom which could be given a primary diagnosis of streptococcal pharyngitis with the differential diagnosis being:

1. Mononucleosis
2. Tonsillitis
3. Peritonsillar abscess
4. Hemophilus influenza epiglottitis

and so on.

The differential diagnosis of CFS must include many disease entities in addition to the Mixed Infection Syndrome (MIS).

In an effort to assist doctors in the differential diagnosis of CFS, the U.S. Center for Disease Control, commonly referred to as the CDC, has developed criteria that they feel are essential for such a diagnosis (Chapter 1.)

The problem for clinicians has been that CFS has been the endpoint diagnosis but without a cause. Elusive, will-o-the-wisp, it's the now you see it; now you don't, magician's dream, and the patient's nightmare. The differential diagnosis of CFS encompasses all the potential causes of chronic fatigue in the individual patient.

We are not saying that these conditions are necessarily part of "the chronic fatigue syndrome." For practical purposes, we shall look at some causes of chronic fatigue which might be of obscure origin yet called CFS until we unearth its real cause. Then if we treat the patients and they get better, then we can call it whatever we like. The patient, however, will spell it r-e-l-i-e-f!

As we write this book, researchers are hard at work to find what could be called a "silver target." The "silver bullet" concept originated with the great microbiologist, Paul Ehrlich. He theorized that there existed the perfect weapon to cure each infection. Ehrlich never really discovered the kind of treatment he sought. Years later, Fleming discovered penicillin, which was probably the first approximation of a silver bullet. For penicillin, there are obvious specific targets like streptococcal pharyngitis (strep throat,) (pneumococcal) pneumonia and, of course, syphilis with which Dr. Ehrlich did so much work. Unfortunately he never had the luxury of using penicillin.

With CFS, we do not yet have a specific target. When and if we discover such a target, the thrust of treatment research will obviously shift to the search for a silver bullet. We cannot design the bullet until we know the target. It is also possible that as you read this book, the single cause of CFS will have been discovered. That will not, however, eliminate all the other causes of chronic fatigue. This chapter addresses the problem of other causes of chronic fatigue which are often called CFS until a true diagnosis becomes clear.

What are the causes of chronic fatigue?

We have included in this book the major differential diagnosis of chronic fatigue as far as we can now deduce. The immune deficiency and consequent Mixed Infection Syndrome (MIS) are the major players which we have addressed up to now. What are other possible contributors?

1. Degenerative disease — Cancer, Heart Disease, Anemia, etc.
2. Anesthesia and surgery
3. Drug reactions (including addiction)
4. Psychological causes (i.e. stress, depression)
5. Fibromyalgia and autoimmunity
6. Low Thyroid and Thyroiditis
7. Adrenal Insufficiency
8. Heavy metal poisoning
9. Obscure malnutrition
10. Chronic exposure to low level electromagnetic radiation
11. Food allergy and The Chemical Hypersensitivity Syndrome

DEGENERATIVE DISEASE—Including arteriosclerotic vascular disease (ASVD), cancer, hypertension, arthritis, multiple sclerosis, etc.

Chronic Fatigue (CF) from degenerative disease floods doctor's offices. At first glance it may appear simple. How obvious! You have arthritis; you suffer fatigue. The same could be said for hardening of the arteries, (arteriosclerotic vascular disease (ASVD)) cancer, and a host of other diseases. We mention this kind of disease for several reasons.

1. The most compelling reasons are coexistence and camouflage. If a patient has cancer, he may not have fatigue from the cancer itself. The cancer may coexist with some hidden infection or some other mysterious cause of CF. The cancer camouflages the other cause. In such a case, the CF is erroneously explained by the cancer and no one looks for other plausible causes. In such a case we have treated patients with our not so specific approach to fatigue. The patients' fatigue may then melt away even though the cancer or other disease remains unchanged. The incidents which baffle are the "incurable" diseases which sometimes resolve themselves. We have seen this with ASVD, arthritis, and many other degenerative diseases. Medically, experts ascribe these cases of disease reversal to "spontaneous regression." This term has no more scientific meaning than "voodoo cure." They both mean essentially, that some unknown force has worked for the patient's betterment. One must acknowledge that there are forces presently unknown which influence biochemistry and health. Moving in the right direction, these forces create health; our job as clinicians is to unmask these hidden energy cures.

2. The second condition which occurs in the CF/degenerative disease connection reverses the situation. In this case the CF manifests clearly, but the degenerative disease remains obscure. Early ASVD and cancer may fool us for fairly long times, sometimes years.

ANEMIA

Some diseases are simple for a doctor to diagnose, but remain undetected because the patient never seeks medical help. Anemia is probably the clearest example. Anemia commonly causes fatigue. The simplest blood test reveals anemia. The specific kind of anemia and specific treatment usually follow with standard medical procedure. The puzzle persists if the fatigue remains after the anemia resolves.

ANESTHESIA and SURGERY

Anesthesia takes surgical patients as close to death as possible without actually killing them. Anesthesiology has become so skilled at this precarious game that rarely do we now have anesthesia deaths. No more do we hear "The operation was a success, but the patient died." That was usually the result of our primitive anesthesia technology. Our modern sophisticated anesthesia rarely kills, but may leave the patient with lasting fatigue. We have observed that many CFS patients date the onset of their CF problem to an operation. With surgery, there are always multiple factors which could explain a person's persistent post operative fatigue:

1. Unless the surgery was purely cosmetic, the patient was suffering from a physical ailment, be it injury, degeneration, cancer, infection, congenital disfigurement etc. Any such ailment may result in persistent post-operative physical or emotional debility.
2. Hidden post-operative infection could also cause persistent problems.
3. Fear and stress of surgery
4. Blood loss
5. Scar tissue and persistent pain
6. Nutrient demands during healing
7. Of course, the anesthesia could explain chronic fatigue. The liver and kidney which detoxify most anesthetics utilize biochemicals comprised of nutrients. In a poorly nourished patient, this could create a sub-clinical malnutrition which could lead to CFS/CF.

As you will see in subsequent chapters, any major demand on the metabolism has the potential to deplete the immune system. Anesthesia is a selective, reversible poison. It puts demands of enormous proportion on the immune defense. In our experience, vitamin A supplements will reverse much of the resulting damage on the immune system. If the patient does not have adequate reserves of vitamin A at the time of surgery, the surgery and anesthesia can easily push the immune system over the edge. Our experience clearly shows that surgery typically suppresses the immune system for about one month.

Our reason for speculating on this unproven idea of post-anesthesia-CFS stems from our experience and that of other physicians who study CFS. Jay Goldstein, M.D.,[1] who specializes in CFS, has observed this to be a common association. We also find that treating such patients intensely with nutrients will often effect a quick recovery.

DRUG REACTIONS

Drugs of both legal and illegal variety may trigger CFS. The metabolism can not read the legal statutes. Medical anesthesia uses drugs which selectively poison the brain until it achieves painless unconsciousness. Anesthesia, therefore, can be used as an illustration of the reaction of the body to drugs in general. Though anesthesia is an extreme example, all drugs are, by definition, selective poisons. Even over-the-counter products function thusly. Aspirin, for example, poisons our ability to feel certain kinds of pain. Prescription drugs, like pain killers and tranquilizers, have many pharmacological properties similar to anesthesia, though not as extreme in normal doses. We all know what over-dosage can do. These drugs in normal dosage generally achieve their therapeutic effect by blocking enzyme systems selectively. Poisons do exactly the same thing, but without the possible therapeutic effect that drugs can achieve. All drugs, therefore, be they called good or bad, selectively poison live tissue. How we use them determines the response of the user, and our attitude about them.

Speaking of attitude, look at morphine and heroin—very similar drugs. Morphine is good because it is legal; heroin is illegal and is bad. They both have great therapeutic powers and, of course, great potential for abuse. Cocaine used for local anesthesia by a physician is good; cocaine sniffed by a "junkie" is bad. Considering the abuses of prescription tranquilizers, sleeping pills, amphetamines, and pain killers, the hazy border between "good" and "bad" drugs can blur to the indistinguishable.

CFS does not distinguish; CFS results. CFS can follow the use of either good or bad drugs in susceptible individuals. The liver and kidney detoxify most of the drugs with biochemical agents produced in the body from nutrients. These organs share this function with the immune system. We could say that drugs compete with the immune system for available nutrients. If we say that our bodies function like a symphony orchestra, any dysfunctional instrument creates discord. Discordant CFS appears when nutrient inadequacy undersupplies the immune system. The principle seems simple.

Drugs, therefore, are poisons that use up nutrients which the immune system requires. If a shortage of nutrients exists, the immune system must compete with the rest of the bodily functions for limited supplies. Something has got to give. The body's defenses will falter when drugs use up available nutrient reserves.

We see this clearly in CFS patients who unwittingly use medications which may harm more than help. Simple culprits like laxatives, aspirin, "cold pills," and certainly many prescription drugs, can contribute to CFS. These medications belong to our way of life. Yet, they can damage and do so insidiously. Sometimes just stopping a "simple" over-the-counter remedy can result in an obvious improvement of the CFS.

Since every drug is a selective poison, it should not surprise us that a number of people suffer fatigue from taking "good" drugs for so long that they forget they are taking something which is basically unnatural and toxic. We have seen many fatigue sufferers who only had to be reminded to stop or change their drugs in order to end their fatigue. The most common drugs which cause fatigue are tranquilizers, followed by antihypertensives. The principle applies. With CFS, consider the patient's drug history. That includes the use of licit and illicit drugs. Illicit drugs are a huge story unto themselves. With or without CFS, drug addiction can lead to an avalanche of health problems which can virtually always includes fatigue. Addiction must be confronted and dealt with—whether or not CFS is present.

Drug dangers, on the other hand, do not mean that we should never use drugs. The work of Jay Goldstein M.D. and others shows that sometimes excellent symptomatic relief of CFS occurs with judicious use of many medical drugs[2]—especially the antidepressants and the anti-ulcer (H2 antagonist) medications. Medicinal drugs are the classical two-edged sword. In one direction they give therapy, but the back edge may damage or destroy. The powerful ability to heal does not occur without risk of damage from most drugs.

We feel that symptoms which defy control with non-drug therapy justify the use of medications. This may occur early in the process when the situation is severe or late in the process when all else fails. In such cases drugs can mitigate the situation greatly and even keep the symptoms under control until the CFS "burns out" or responds to treatment such as we prescribe.

PSYCHOLOGICAL CAUSES

We squeeze this category in a seemingly inconsequential slot in our book. Since depression and stress have received the most blame in CFS, we thought to defuse this misconception by deliberately hiding it in the middle of a chapter. We will not dwell on them. The standard medical belief system already credits them with too much power in CFS.

We should observe that stress and depression result from CFS more than they cause it. The most compelling evidence comes from the patient's history. Most of them lived well adjusted, ambitious lives before being struck with their disease; the disease then depressed them. Illness often leads to reactive depression; the reactive depression of CFS mirrors that of many more "respectable" diseases like heart attacks and cancer. Depression after a heart attack or a broken leg does not surprise anyone. The mysterious nature of CFS confounds our ability to see that the depression is reactive and not causative.

Reactive depression differs from "primary depression" in important ways. Most obviously, the depressed CFS patient hungers for return of health and manifests a powerful ambition frustrated by CFS. Most primary depressed patients do not or cannot exhibit such concern. They barely remember their ambition and zest for life. True, there are many similarities, but the depression of the CFS patient follows the illness, while the primary depression precedes it. In most of our CFS patients, the depression clearly follows the illness. Recall the case report on J.S. the businessman with depression caused by a parasite which we discussed in Chapter 5? He had no depression until he caught dysentary. Additionally, recent work has shown that a relatively new kind of brain scan called SPECT (Single Photo Emission Computerized Tomography) shows a definite decrease in blood perfusion in CFS patients. This perfusion defect is different from that which is found in depressed patients. This finding plus psychological testing is helping now to distinguish CFS from depression and psychosomatic disease (see appendix).

Stress, on the other hand, often participates in the early stages of CFS. The patient's history may include a major life crisis such as a divorce or business problem. Sometimes patients suffer from overachievement or get overwhelmed by their self-imposed heavy schedules. Such schedules burden these CFS people, but are their schedules worse those than those of many modern people without CFS? We ponder the question of whether the so-called "heavy schedules" truly exceed the norm. Statistics, after all, can mislead. We could, for example make a case against tooth brushing by noting that almost 100% of CFS victims brush their teeth daily. When we question healthy people in today's society, their stress levels often equal those of patients who fall prey to CFS.

Stress makes every disease worse, and every disease increases the stress response. Hans Selye, the great medical researcher, first defined biological stress as "The non-specific response of the body to any demand put upon it."[3] We all put enormous emotional and physical demands on our bodies. How our bodies respond depends on our emotional and physical reserve. If we have inadequate reserves, we fail to cope. The immune system weakens; infection soon follows. We do not doubt that undue emotional demand will damage the immune system. We recognize that the mind and spirit must heal to have vibrant health. We wish to keep it all in perspective. The total role stress and depression play in CFS still eludes us. The main message, as we see it, is to respect both the body and the mind. Do not treat one with the other. In Chapter 10 we provide a simple approach to stress management.

We need to understand stress in the framework of CFS. Stress no doubt can trigger CFS, and CFS, in turn, raises stress. This vicious cycle influences our treatment imperative which deals with stress in several ways. When appropriate, we first educate the patient on the causes and background of stress. We then suggest possible methods of dealing with the stress depending on the patient's needs and preferences. Though everybody talks about stress as some sort of magic key to CFS, defining and, more importantly, solving stress still stymies most people. In our practice, we have evolved a pragmatic solution to the stress component of CFS. In some patients, we use a self–awareness technique which we have developed. In others, we suggest some of the commonly used approaches such as lifestyle changes, relaxation exercises, therapeutic confrontation of day to day problems, and the nutrients and herbs which help reduce the stress response. We begin by defining stress.

What is stress? Aside from being one of the medical catch words of the eighties, most people—even many professionals—have never heard the definition. Defining stress is the beginning of mastering it.

As we have said, Hans Selye M.D., in the 1930's, defined stress. He observed it in laboratory mice. He put them in water, and they swam until they drowned. The animal rights activists, today, would probably drown Hans Selye for such inhumane treatment of mice. But even today there may not be any better way of discovering stress and its effects. Selye examined the drowned mice and found two organ systems were severely depleted by this prolonged physically and mentally demanding death. The adrenal glands, which sit on top of the kidneys, and the thymus gland, which rests behind the breast bone, were blanched and swollen in these animals. That discovery launched a half century of study of the functional importance of these two organs which are vital to the function of our immune system, as well as integral parts of our endocrine system. Selye made this important discovery. Moreover, he conceptualized stress and defined it as (We repeat.), ***"The non–specific response of the body to any demand made upon it."***

This definition includes any simple demand such as breathing or eating. Selye, therefore, postulated that the stress that causes damage should be called distress. In common usage, we all use "stress" as meaning distress. We will stick to that convention in our discussion of stress.

Selye's stress concept clearly includes the stress that influences CFS. Many doctors attribute CFS to stress alone. We, on the other hand, feel that stress plays a role in CFS, but is not usually the main character. Stress from many different demands may overwhelm the immune system which then allows infection or some other metabolic problem to intervene. There may also be a vicious cycle where CFS causes stress which in turn further weakens the immune system leading to more disease and more stress. It quickly becomes a chicken-or-the-egg proposition. Regardless of which started the cycle, we must deal with the stress as well as the immune and infectious parts of the problem.

When Selye began his work, there was no word in biology for the phenomenon which he observed. Selye borrowed the word, stress, from engineering; he never saw fit to return it. Selye saw this drastic response which was non-specific. No matter what kind of demand he put on the mice, their stress response was the same.

Selye described the stress response in three stages. He called it the General Adaptation Syndrome (G.A.S.). The G.A.S. consists of:

1. Alarm Reaction: Characteristic body changes [increased pulse, blood pressure, sweating, etc.] ——> Diminished resistance [Susceptibility to infection? immune system weakened — Obviously nervous and "stressed"]. Death may result.
2. Stage of Resistance: Adaptation to continued stress with outward disappearance of signs of alarm [Coping, compensating; outwardly in control as the body invests resources in developing resistance to the stress.]
3. Stage of Exhaustion: Continued exposure leads to overwhelm of the resistance and the alarm reaction reappears [exhausted, collapsing, "stressed-out" and vulnerable to more serious and persistent infection]. Selye says the ultimate result is irreversible damage and even death.

Humans have many causes of stress. Elsewhere in the book we have talked about nutrient deficiency, toxicity from pollution, toxicity from licit and illicit drugs, physical injury, infection, and, the most obvious cause, emotional upset. All of these demands easily fit into the vicious cycle of CFS and MIS. Stress and disease play off each other.

Most people think of stress as coming from the mind and from external sources. Remember, Selye defined stress as a *response* of the *body* (not the mind) to any *demand* (external or internal). The key words are response, body, and demand. The mind can trigger a stress response and recognize it, but the brain is not the major response organ. Selye's work indicates that the adrenal and thymus glands occupy that position. New discoveries in neurotransmitter physiology may change that concept in the near future, but for now we will work with Selye's classical discoveries.

It may be that stress will ultimately turn out to be the major psychological factor in CFS. It may turn out to be the most important of all factors, considering its links with the immune system and all the damage it can do there.

In the appendix, we include some further discussion of the nature of stress and an outline of the Stress Mastery tape which we sometimes recommend to our patients.

FIBROMYALGIA

Fibromyalgia is a condition that mimics CFS and which many people think may be CFS in disguise. This perplexing condition, which is often also called "fibrositis," involves many of the same dread symptoms seen in CFS: overwhelming and persistent fatigue, headache and diffuse muscle aches and pains, poor memory and concentration, numbness, tingling and burning sensations of the hands and feet and a nagging sleep disorder. In fibromyalgia, however, there is more of an emphasis on disabling muscle pain and tenderness than in CFS. Physical examination reveals widespread tender points which are diagnostic of this condition.

The striking similarity between fibromyalgia and CFS cannot be ignored. Recent studies show that a majority of CFS patients fulfill the tender point criteria for the diagnosis of fibromyalgia. In some studies, upwards of 80% of CFS patients are said to have fibromyalgia.

Many experts believe that fibromyalgia is due to the chronic stress of an underlying emotional disorder. Some patient surveys find upwards of 90% of fibromyalgia patients to be suffering from assorted psychoneuroses. The course of this disease is every bit as unrelenting and disabling as CFS. There is no simple or effective treatment for it.

Pain control is frustrating because the usual analgesics do not work very well. An antidepressant drug known as "doxepin" has been especially helpful in relieving aches and pains and correcting the sleep disorder.

LOW THYROID AND THYROIDITIS

Low thyroid conditions comprise a significant source of chronic fatigue. Hypothyroidism primarily affects women and tends to worsen with age. We also feel that many people with *marginal* hypothyroidism remain undiagnosed. Thyroid hormone controls our metabolism (the rate at which our cells burn oxygen and fuel). A person with a low thyroid condition will tend to have an overall sluggish metabolism which can manifest itself in a variety of ways that may mimic CFS:

1. Fatigue, which tends to be worse upon awakening in the morning and may improve late at night. Many of our low thyroid patients tell us that they only "get going" after ten P.M.
2. Cold intolerance which includes cold feet and hands and a tendency to wear more clothing than others.
3. Easy weight gain and difficulty losing weight on a conventional low calorie weight loss diet.
4. Chronic constipation
5. Low blood pressure
6. Dry skin
7. Hair thinning and hair loss
8. Heavy and irregular menstrual periods
9. Depression. In this regard, it is interesting that even low doses of thyroid hormone may potentiate the action of antidepressant medication.
10. Inability to think clearly
11. Low blood sugar and a craving for carbohydrates.

Fatigue and coldness are the most common low thyroid afflictions. However, any combination of the above listed symptoms can occur with this condition.

How does hypothyroidism differ from CFS? The CFS patient is not only tired but usually has malaise (sick feeling), fever and body aches. There is a thyroid dysfunction that does cause flu-like symptoms. This is called "Hashimoto thyroiditis," an autoimmune disease that predominates in women by a ratio of almost ten to one. The incidence of this condition is rising for unknown reasons. The incidence of thyroiditis appears to be higher in CFS patients than in the general population. It is said to afflict about 6% of American women; 10% to 15% more closely approximates our female patients. Why the disparity? Physicians rarely discover the presence of thyroiditis because the routine thyroid blood test does not diagnose it. Thyroiditis requires a specific blood assay. We recommend using only an RIA (radioactive iodine) assay for anti-thyroid microsomal and thyroglobulin antibodies. More controversial than the diagnosis is the treatment of thyroiditis. Most conventional medical doctors observe the condition and treat the disorder with thyroid hormone only if the patient underproduces thyroid hormone. A new tide of opinion favors treatment with thyroid hormone even if blood thyroid hormone levels are normal, because thyroid hormone tends to thwart the immune attack against the gland.

Obviously, if one misses the obscure diagnoses of hypothyroidism or thyroiditis, one may mistake the problem for CFS.

ADRENAL INSUFFICIENCY

The adrenal glands protect us against stress and inflammation. These almond sized glands have a central core called the medulla and a thin outer layer called the adrenal cortex, which produces cortisol, a steroid hormone that flows in response to stress. Stress comes from many sources, which can be either physical or emotional. For example, anxiety and depression create stress in the body. Physical trauma from accidents, surgery or burns may provoke extreme stress. Infections also stress us, whether they are acute and short-lived like a head cold or prolonged—like CFS. In all of these cases, the body pours out cortisol to soften the blows and prevent the attendant pain, tenderness, swelling and fever.

Since its discovery some fifty years ago, cortisol and its analogues have gained increasing prominence in the treatment of autoimmune diseases, allergies, asthma and athletic injuries. Over the years, researchers have developed powerful synthetic forms of these steroids with stronger anti-inflammatory effects. When first introduced, these synthetic hormones were hailed as wonder drugs. Unfortunately, in continued high doses, these "corticosteroids" cause adverse side effects, which include depression, fluid retention, high blood pressure, bone loss, gastrointestinal ulcers, bleeding disorders, and many other toxicities.

CFS, which may go on for years, puts relentless strain on the adrenal glands. Theoretically, chronic stress can deplete the adrenal glands to the point of "adrenal exhaustion." The nutritional and medicinal management of this adrenal exhaustion can make a huge difference in how a CFS patient ultimately responds.

THE ADRENAL LOWS

Adrenal insufficiency may cause a myriad of lows:

- low blood sugar
- low blood pressure
- low energy and endurance
- low mental capacity
- low body temperature
- low body weight
- low feeling of well-being—This may explain the "high" some people get with steroid treatment.

Beyond adrenal lows, is "Addison's Disease," the severe adrenal insufficiency which results from the actual destruction of the adrenal glands. This major disease is usually permanent, and occurs when cancer, or an infection like tuberculosis, invades and destroys the glands. A relatively simple blood test can diagnose it rather quickly. Conversely, the adrenal "weakness" that accompanies chronic stress, is a marginal and temporary insufficiency, much more difficult to diagnose. We ascertain this marginal adrenal insufficiency by clinical suspicion rather than solid laboratory evidence. The so-called stressed out adrenal gland may enlarge a bit, but otherwise it appears structurally sound, and usually produces normal blood levels of cortisol. How then can we detect adrenal stress? A book entitled *Safe Uses of Cortisone* by Dr. William Jefferies, a prominent endocrinologist, clarifies the nature of adrenal stress and how to test for it.

Dr. Jefferies concludes that "weak" adrenal glands can supply adequate cortisol when the body suffers little stress. Therefore, single determinations of blood cortisol in a person with marginal adrenal insufficiency are usually normal. However, expose this same person to a major stressful event, and the adrenals may flunk the challenge due to their low reserve of steroid hormones.

In the doctor's office, the ACTH stimulation test can detect the adrenal "blahs." ACTH is the pituitary hormone that specifically stimulates the adrenal glands to secrete cortisol. By a simple intramuscular injection, ACTH can approximate the action of the pituitary control of the adrenal cortex. Appropriate measurements of blood levels of cortisol before and after the injection can reveal the status of the adrenal reserve. The usual procedure is to obtain a baseline blood level of cortisol and immediately give an injection of ACTH. Thirty minutes later, we draw a second sample and measure for cortisol which should be at least double above the baseline level to reach a satisfactory range. Weak adrenals fail the test. This adrenal situation pertains mightily to CFS and CF. We suspect that a majority of such patients have significant exhaustion of adrenal reserve.

One theoretical solution to the problem of adrenal exhaustion is intravenous (IV) Adrenal Cortical Extract (ACE): The story of ACE in the United States is strange. The use of ACE dates back to the 1930's during a time at which it was the treatment of choice for Addison's disease (failure of the adrenal gland). Such medical luminaries as George Thorne, M.D., the eminent endocrinologist and Chief of Medicine at Harvard Medical School, studied it extensively. Dr. Thorne was a leading proponent of ACE until cortisone was discovered and became more favored by the American medical community. ACE then evolved into a medical niche which seemed to make it more of a nutrient than a drug. It is an extract of beef adrenal glands and therefore has, in principle, more similarity to nutritional liver shots than it does to synthetically produced cortisone. It was widely used in the USA until the late 1970's when the U.S. Food and Drug Administration (US FDA) made the puzzling ruling forbidding its manufacture. The FDA claimed that ACE was obsolete; there was never a question of its safety, and its effectiveness was still the same. It was just weaker than the more recent synthetic cortisone—therefore, "obsolete." ACE is still used widely in many countries of the world. In France and Switzerland, for example, one can purchase ACE of high quality over the counter—without a prescription. In America, it is perfectly safe and legal to use; it just cannot be manufactured here!

The purpose in mentioning this somewhat controversial substance is its theoretical usefulness in stressful conditions, possibly including CFS. There are anecdotal reports from Europe, of patients who are "stressed-out" to such a degree that they could barely function. These people claim to feel instantly renewed when given ACE. It has potential uses in allergy and other immune imbalances. Hopefully, ACE will someday be readily available again in the U.S.

HEAVY METAL POISONING

Are we all lead poisoned? Are we mercury poisoned? What about other toxic metals?

Claire Patterson, Ph.D., the highly esteemed geologist at the California Institute of Technology in Pasadena, California, says that all modern-living people are sub-clinically lead poisoned. Dr. Patterson has been studying lead levels around the world and in humans for about three decades. He has discovered that the average civilized human now has a body burden of lead that is about 1000 times greater than people living 500 years ago.[4] Patterson further notes that our burden of lead approximates the level which existed in ancient Rome; this level, he postulates, is just below the modern level that the medical community acknowledges to be lead poisoning. This sub-clinical state of lead toxicity affects vast numbers of unsuspecting victims worldwide. When we combine this information with the study by the U.S. Environmental Protection Agency (EPA) which calculates the massive medical cost estimated to result from the overburden of lead in a segment of the United States population, we have reason to suspect lead as a hidden cause of many diseases and symptom complexes in our modern populations.[5] This health problem, which lead presents politically and demographically, would need more than all the health resources of every government in the world, if the world decided to correct it. We, as doctors and individuals, can take steps to help ourselves and not count on the authorities.

What has this to do with CFS? Maybe nothing directly. There are, however, certain realities about CF and the toxicity of heavy metals which means that we have to explore the connection. Lead or other metal toxicities must be part of the differential diagnosis.

Fatigue and immune suppression can result from low grade chronic toxicity to lead and other heavy metals such as cadmium or mercury. Since most doctors have no notion of the facts about lead toxicity, they have no suspicion of it when a patient presents with CFS. If lead happens to be the cause of CF in a patient, it could look like CFS, and it will not be discovered accidentally. No doctor will just stumble onto it. It takes specific tests and deliberate consideration to diagnose sub-clinical lead poisoning. Because of the inadequacy of our present testing technology, sometimes the only way to diagnose lead toxicity is with a therapeutic trial. Treat the CF as if it were caused by lead poisoning, even if the tests are not conclusive. If the patient responds favorably to the therapeutic trial, that may be presumptive evidence that lead is the problem. The more specific the treatment in a therapeutic trial, the more conclusive is the diagnostic evidence. The treatment of lead poisoning is not specific for lead per se, but it is rather specific for toxic metals as discussed above.

EDTA (ethylene diamine tetra acetic acid) is the major drug treatment for lead poisoning. It is a synthetic amino acid (and therefore in some ways, more like a food than a drug,) which binds heavy metals like lead, cadmium, mercury, nickel, arsenic, etc., and takes them into solution in the blood from whence the kidneys excrete them. This process, then, is not specific for lead. It works on many toxic metals. It also removes from the body some worthwhile nutritional minerals like zinc, calcium, magnesium, selenium, etc.

EDTA is also used therapeutically to remove excess calcium which is a nutrient which may easily assume a toxic role when it gets in the wrong place in the body or becomes excessive in the right place. It is also possible that a barely measurable imbalance of calcium and magnesium in the cells can cause fatigue of obscure origin, but with that we digress too far for this discussion, except to emphasize how non-specific EDTA is for removing lead.

The American College of Advancement in Medicine (ACAM)[6] lists among its members hundreds of physicians who use EDTA for various purposes. EDTA therapy benefits patients in many ways. Although it primarily reverses lead or calcium toxicity medically, ACAM doctors have for over two decades treated vascular conditions with EDTA. This use of EDTA has remained controversial, although there is increasing evidence world-wide that this EDTA therapy reverses certain vascular diseases of the heart, head and limbs. ACAM doctors have reportedly treated over one half million people for these conditions.

How does this pertain to CFS? As one might imagine, vascular patients are generally older, and in the U.S., usually of Medicare age. Many older patients complain of fatigue. Fatigue looms large in geriatrics. No one pays much attention to it. Doctors, bystanders, and victims all consider it an inevitable part of aging. It may not be! A significant number, perhaps 25%, of fatigued geriatric patients getting EDTA treatment for vascular diseases, get remarkable relief of their fatigue and a concomitant sense of well being. We have seen this happen also in younger patients with fatigue, to whom we have given therapeutic trials of EDTA on the chance that they cannot handle the body burden of lead that typifies our modern world population. Remember that individuals have a wide spectrum of response to any offending agent such as lead. Because of this individual variation, dramatic reversals of fatigue syndrome have occurred in a small but significant percentage of CFS patients of all ages — when treated with EDTA.

CASE REPORT

Cassie, an attractive, charming, thirty-two year old, mother of two children and a legal secretary, suffered with fatigue and muscle pain for seventeen years. She could only function at about one half of her expected work output. She had continued muscle pain and tenderness especially after exercise. She had bouts of depression and self-described "spaciness." She also suffered frequent sore throats and fevers. Cassie had visited numerous physicians with little benefit over the years. She tried numerous therapies, including diet, antidepressants, H2 antagonists, nutritional supplements, injections of homeopathic remedies, antibiotics, various anti-candida medications, infusions of intravenous vitamins, and infusions of intravenous oxidative therapy from hydrogen peroxide. Nothing worked. After failing with several of our more standard approaches, we tried a small dose of EDTA intravenously. EDTA chelates (binds to) heavy metals such as lead and cadmium. The EDTA then puts the toxic metal into solution so that it can be excreted by the kidneys. After Cassie's first intravenous EDTA infusion, she experienced an immediate relief of symptoms which lasted for about eight days. Laboratory examination of a twenty-four hour urine specimen revealed increased levels of lead in the urine after chelation therapy, indicating an increased body burden of sequestered lead which was extracted by the chelation. A second intravenous chelation with EDTA produced the same improved symptoms for several days longer. Each subsequent treatment gave increasingly longer lasting results, until Cassie considered herself cured. It took about ten treatments.

It is difficult to draw a certain conclusion from this case. Without going into the multitude of possible reasons for her positive response, suffice it to say that the patient's long standing fatigue scattered to the winds following treatment. Lead removal explains the result logically. EDTA, however, is not specific for lead. Other toxic metals such as cadmium, arsenic, mercury, etc. could also bind with EDTA and leave the body with less of a total toxic burden. Remember that heavy metals also poison the immune system. We could postulate that the reason viruses, yeast, parasites and bacteria sometimes run wild in some CFS victims, hinges on their total toxic metal levels. That could explain some of the mysterious cases of CFS.

The question often arises: "If we are all lead poisoned, why are we all not sick? How come we all do not have CFS or worse?" We answer that biological individuality applies to low grade lead poisoning as well as every other human and animal species trait. DDT did not kill all the boll weevils. Penicillin did not kill all the streptococci. Bubonic plague did not kill everyone in medieval Europe. Species have a range of genetic traits which includes giving certain individuals resistance to various threats such as infection or lead poisoning. We affirm that we must look at individual CFS patients with the intention of seeking the possible cause and converting the frustrating CFS into a curable CF. We desire further research by the medical community to create standardized and sufficient procedures to resolve this problem.

This book would expand into volumes of encyclopedic length if we went into full detail on lead and other heavy metals worth considering in the differential diagnosis of CFS. However, we will address those items which we feel are important causes of CF, understanding that we must limit ourselves to less detail.

OTHER TOXIC HEAVY METALS

CADMIUM

What other toxic metals might be considered in the CFS picture? Take cadmium, for example, a highly toxic metal known to cause hypertension[7] and other diseases. It can also cause profound effects on immune cells. Cadmium is particularly noteworthy as a toxic metal since it increases the toxicity of not only most other toxic metals, but of many immune suppressing chemicals. The major source of cadmium is from cigarette smoke. It is found in both the cigarette's paper and in the tobacco leaf, hence "side-stream" tobacco source is potentially a source of toxic levels of cadmium in non-smokers. Carpets in many homes and businesses have a rubber backing which contains cadmium added to it to harden the rubber. Automobile tires contain this metal for the same reason. Many incinerators are being recognized as sources of cadmium toxicity because cadmium has a low melting point compared to most metals. These incinerators do not have scrubbers that are capable of preventing this highly toxic metal from becoming airborne. When combined with copper or chlorinated compounds non-toxic doses of cadmium can become highly toxic. *Cadmium is the most potent immune modulator among the toxic metals,* and is capable of causing several autoimmune disorders. Since mercury also can cause autoimmune disorders and impair immune function, it is certainly worth discussing.

MERCURY

Mercury invades the central nervous system, causing neurologic dysfunction. It also invades the kidneys and other organ systems as discovered at autopsy. For 150 years, dentists have used mercury-silver amalgams to fill our decayed teeth. There are entire books devoted to this volatile and urgent subject, such as *It's All In Your Head* by Hal Huggins, D.D.S.[8]

We suspect that many patients with CFS have too much mercury in their body. Many foreward thinking dentists now remove the amalgams from patients with evidence of mercury toxicity causing fatigue. Removing the amalgams often seems to correct CF. Once again, this is difficult to prove and hotly controversial. Mercury also finds its way to the top of the ocean food chain. Large fish, such as tuna, swordfish, shark, salmon, and large lobsters carry mercury into our bodies through the diet. For most of us, eating these foods moderately, perhaps twice weekly, poses no threat. Some people who consume such fish daily may accumulate toxic levels of mercury. We observed a case of a man who ate three cans of tuna daily for years. His laboratory analysis for heavy metals showed mercury at astronomical numbers. He suffered significant neurologic deficit, and was barely able to continue to work. By stopping the tuna intake and getting a course of chelation with the drug BAL, a chelating agent that is more specific for mercury, the patient achieved vast improvement. In early 1991, the popular TV magazine, *60 Minutes*, stirred further controversy by revealing increasing world-wide evidence indicating that mercury-silver amalgams may be causing serious damage to many patients afflicted with various central nervous system disorders, including multiple sclerosis. These contentions were hotly rejected by a spokesperson for the American Dental Association (ADA). However, even more recently Hal Huggins, D.D.S. has published that a number of major industrial nations such Sweden, Japan, and Germany are taking steps toward reducing or eliminating mercury in all fillings, particularly in females of child-bearing age.

ALUMINUM

Aluminum comprises about 8% of the Earth's crust and structures much of our mechanized world. The food industry and drug industry both use aluminum widely. Research increasingly associates the presence of excessive levels of aluminum in the brains of patients with the dementia known as Alzheimer's disease. This brain destroyer of a huge percentage of our elderly population may exist in a lesser state in people of all ages who have been labeled CFS. This is still highly speculative, but worth mentioning. When our technology for measuring aluminum becomes adequate, we may find yet another piece of the CFS/CF puzzle. Aluminum absorbs into the body much more readily than formerly believed. Its aborption and consequent danger increases with simple daily foods like orange juice which contains citric acid. Citric acid insidiously increases the intestinal absorption of aluminum. Medicinal aluminum in antacids has caused encephalopathy (brain toxicity) in patients on renal dialysis. Powdered underarm deordorants with aluminum is another suspected common source of this toxic metal. The spray from such powders has been found to be absorbed through the sinus passages almost directly into the brain. Whether, and how, aluminum is involved in chronic fatigue and CFS continues to be studied, but since it is a known neurotoxin, it may be essential in determining the differential diagnosis of CF/CFS.

It behooves us to know that the result of any acute or chronic exposure to toxic metals may be subtle. Artists with their paints and clays and metals risk accumulation of toxins. Plumbers, machinists, gardeners, mechanics, drivers, painters, farmers, and those in many other occupations suffer the risks of all kinds of metal toxins. Of course, the most insidious danger is just what is in our polluted environments. Many individuals will not tolerate typical levels of modern toxicity. We all need to increase our vigilance in these areas; we hope that more doctors will consider these metals in their patient's histories.

OBSCURE MALNUTRITION

The idea of possible post-surgical malnutrition leads us to a greater and more important likelihood. It may well be that most of the conventionally nourished people in the civilized world, are in reality undernourished. This flies in the face of all the scientific claims of official agencies like the U.S. FDA that claimed otherwise throughout the 1980's. According to the FDA, we are all fully nourished as long as we eat the amounts of nutrients which the government has determined that we need. The U.S. RDA's (Recommended Daily Allowances) have been politically determined to some degree for many years, since they emphasize minimal nutrient requirements in humans, not optimal levels. RDA's fail as a true indication of nutrient content needs; they do not account for the diminished nutrition of the actual food that we consume. The RDA considers nutrient levels in an idealized food supply. Most of the food which finally gets to our plates has traveled through a maze of changes that affect nutrient levels. From the onset of food production, which begins with the seed, to the last moment when our intestines begin to absorb the digested foodstuff into our bloodstreams, anti-nutritional influences can substantially damage the nutrient content of the food.

Someone once said that "Land that makes money cannot make food." That may be an exaggeration, but there certainly is some truth to this statement today. The production of food often begins on soil that is overused and heavily dependent on chemical fertilizers and herbicides. Today the act of farming strays incredibly far from ancesteral methods of gathering food in dense forests, jungles, or on prairie fields. Modern agri-business practices require that a farmer harvest some crops before they properly ripen to prevent premature spoilage in our market places. For a number of foods, ripening on the vine improves their nutrient content. Vitamin C in oranges, for example, is almost non-existent until ripened. Unripe oranges need artificial coloring and artificial agents to ripen them and make them presentable to the consumer. We all accept as ordinary the standard food processes of refrigeration, freezing, canning, boxing, packaging, dehydrating, reconstituting, irradiating, and the addition of preservatives, colors, artificial flavors, softeners, hardeners, emulsifiers, fragrances. All of these processes damage the nutrition of the food. Add to this unintentional contaminants, some of which we discussed at the beginning of the chapter: miniscule (but significant?) amounts of lead, other heavy metals, petrochemicals, rodent droppings, mold, bacteria, insects, and more, can reach our plates. We have every reason to suspect malnutrition. This panoply of agricultural and food industry manipulation tends to diminish our food supplies nutritional value in ways as yet not fully understood or appreciated.

In addition to certain toxins already mentioned in this chapter, we must consider other stresses. Certainly stress from emotional tensions, excess noise pollution, chronic low level electromagnetic radiation exposure and drug misuse, are examples of stresses that can increase our nutritional needs or modify our immune system.

Whatever the reasons, the majority of us seem to require nutritional supplementation beyond that supplied by our diets. This is especially true with aging, and in the prevention of certain degenerative diseases. Imagine—a majority of dieticians (who universally claim our diet is adequate) polled about their supplement intake report taking vitamin/mineral supplements. Experientially we see in our practice CFS patients who sometimes respond dramatically to nutritional supplementation. It well may be that many fatigue problems actually represent a gradual continuum of declining nutritional status culminating for some as CFS. There is no disputing that our body's nutrient levels influence our physiology at all levels and to various degrees. The testing of nutritional status again is esoteric, expensive, and woefully inadequate. We, therefore, have learned to rely on the therapeutic trial model for safety and economic reasons.

If a patient with fatigue and depression, especially one who has tried numerous medical therapies with unsuccessful results, recovers quickly and decisively on just nutrient supplements, it is likely to mean one of four things.

1. It was a placebo effect. About 40% of people are placebo responders, but placebo responders generally lose the place-

bo effect within a few months as the sham treatment continues.

2. It was coincidental. The condition reached its readiness to resolve spontaneously, and the therapy happened to start at that opportune time.
3. It was the nutritional supplementation. The patient truly lacked adequate levels of certain nutrients, and in the absence of frank nutritional deficiency, probably suffered from a sub-clinical deficiency. The nutritional therapy corrected this need, restoring the body to a homeostatic level of good health.
4. Our nutritional counseling effectively modified the patients diet so that the elimination of poor nutritional foods, and their substitution with nutritionally dense and healthier foodstuffs, resulted in an overall physical and emotional improvement.

Placebo and coincidence do not bear the test of time. If a patient responds well to nutritional therapy and the fatigue dissipates, we usually reduce the nutritional therapy, observe the response, and restart it if necessary. If the patient loses the benefit and then regains it with the restart of the therapy, presumably some beneficial effect of nutrients did occur. This sequence virtually eliminates coincidence as a cause and argues against placebo. Placebo tends to lose its effect as time goes on and does not generally return with the same vigor when restarted. Nutritional therapy, on the other hand, gets better and better as the patient gets replenished. In our experience, the patient needs less nutrition as the therapy goes on. We explain this phenomenon as the result of restoration of depleted body stores.

We have literally thousands of cases of clear response to nutritional counseling and/or nutritional supplementation. One of our favorite cases, presenting as fatigue, illustrates that depression might easily be mistaken for the cause of CF, when malnutrition is the real culprit.

CASE HISTORY

Ralph was a thirty-six year old school teacher with two children and a lovely devoted wife. He preferred working as a free lance artist on stained class and sculpture. He had been too tired, confused, anxious and depressed to continue in his artistic enterprise. He had recurrent sore throats, muscle aches and increasing fears about his sanity and his ability to continue to function as a father and provider. He had been diagnosed as having a neurosis or possibly a reactive depression. He was advised to start psychotherapy and anti-depressant drugs.

He also had financial problems. His insurance would cover standard medical care with psychiatry and medications, but would not cover any nutritional therapy or uncoventional tests. We decided that he had a history which could be explained by obscure malnutrition, and we started him on our simple Basic Therapeutic Diet (see Chapter 10), and relatively inexpensive supplements consisting of desiccated liver capsules and our multiple vitamin and mineral formulation. Initially, we used fairly high doses. We also gave him several intramuscular injections ("butt shots") of certain vitamins and a liver extract. Ralph responded almost immediately. In three days, there was clear improvement. In a week, his depression was virtually gone and his energy was returning to normal. His gratitude and glee at his recovery satisfied in us all those slightly corny, almost forgotten motives that entice students into medical school. Everyone in our office who knew him and his predicament shared his joy. Ralph felt he was rescued from being institutionalized and returned from the dead.

Despite all the joy, Ralph was not all the way out of the woods. He improved continuously for some weeks, only to relapse resoundingly as he let his diet discipline slip away. When he restored himself to the program, he returned to the healing path. Ralph only used diet and nutrient supplements, both oral and by injection. He never took antidepressant drugs or psychotherapy.

This case illustrates the potential power of nutrition in CFS. Was this patient suffering CFS? He could easily have been diagnosed as such. Was Ralph just CF from nutritional needs or was he just suffering a primary depression? If he was not suffering malnutritive dysfunction, then it must have been a placebo-responding emotional dysfunction.

Too many doctors give too little attention to the role of nutrition in many disease states, including CFS.[9] It comes as no surprise to those of us who have studied the role of nutrition in medicine to see the excellent response of a CFS patient to proper nutritional management.

LOW LEVEL ELECTROMAGNETIC RADIATION AND OTHER UNSEEN ENERGY FORCES

If we were to approach CFS from the atomic and molecular level, we could easily drive ourselves crazy. Certainly, every function in the body ultimately occurs at the atomic or sub-atomic level. We understand many of these energies, while much of this type of energy still defies scientific explanation. Even those which we understand are still only understood at relatively superficial levels.

There are many reports about the importance of various forms of low level electromagnetic energy. Robert Becker, in the book *The Body Electric*, and John Ott, in his series on light and low level electromagnetic radiation in the *International Journal of Biosocial and Medical Research*, have both cautioned us to consider the potential dangers of such common electromagnetic sources as a simple electric blanket, a kitchen microwave oven, or a computer terminal.

Of even greater significance may be the electric fields emanating from high intensity power lines. Current research at best confuses the problem, but we have seen at least one patient whose CFS seemed related to her moving to a house located near high tension electrical power lines.

Computer terminal radiation also concerns many scientists who have measured energies that may harm the operator of the terminal. At best, the radiation emitted by the cathode ray tube has *low* toxicity. Few people doubt that there is toxicity. What effect such exposure has over time is still being researched. Microwaves, home TV's, electric alarm clocks, atomic energy generating medical x-rays, are just some of the examples of objects that might suppress the immune system of vulnerable people.

When it comes to radiation sources, we would suggest that you avoid or reduce your exposure to any known potentially harmful radiation source. For example, never sit closer to a TV or a computer terminal than you must.

There is also good evidence that changes in ions in the air we breath can influence the levels of neurotransmitters in the brain affecting mood states in susceptible people. Three decades of studies carried out by Dr. Felix Sulman at Hadassah University Medical Center in Jerusalem has established that approximately one half of the human population can be adversely affected by the changes in the ratios of negative and positive ions in our atmosphere. When too many positive ions are generated in the air we breath, an exhaustion syndrome can develop which is characterized by slowed reactions, reduced acuity, lethargy, sleepiness, an inability to concentrate, apathy, depression, a sense of exhaustion, mental confusion, physical fatigue, sluggish circulation, and poor muscular coordination. The book, *The Ion Controversy: A Scientific Appraisal*, by Charles Wallach, discusses this problem in detail. If you suspect that the periodic changes in ion ratios might be responsible for your CF, consider purchasing a negative ion generator. Negative ion generators create fields of negative ions to combat the adverse effects of increased positive ion levels. A number of patients have reported on the beneficial effects of these devices. We mention this only because some report dramatic improvements.

FOOD ALLERGY AND THE CHEMICAL HYPERSENSITIVITY SYNDROME

It is easy to spot the itchy, watery eyes, sneezing and runny nose of an airborne allergy attack. These reactions are obvious and occur almost immediately after inhaling the dust, mold or pollen to which one is sensitive. Food allergies are different! The majority of food reactions commence hours to days after eating a food. This delay masks the connection between cause and effect and is the main reason that food allergies elude detection.

Other factors make it even harder to pin down the diagnosis: food allergies can be caused by a wide variety of foods and can occur both indoors and outdoors at any time of year. Food reactions are not limited to the airborne allergic triad of eyes, ears, and nose—but can also affect the skin, muscles, joints, digestive and urinary tracts, and the brain.

The food immune scenario is more complex than its airborne counterpart. Airborne allergies are caused by one basic reaction: the release of histamine and other chemical mediators from "mast cells" which have been coated by IgE antibodies which are targeted to bind to one specific type of allergen. In contrast, there are many possible causes for food allergy. The IgE antibody participates in only about 10% of food reactions, but these can be abrupt and serious resulting in eczema, hives and even life-threatening swelling of the lips and tongue. Shellfish and nuts cause most IgE food reactions. There is a serious rift in the medical community as to whether the other 90% of food reactions even exist! Most allergists put their stock solely in the IgE camp. Environmental allergists and ear, nose, throat specialists have dramatically expanded the range of food allergy research. They believe that IgG, by far the most prevalent of all circulating antibodies, plays the predominant role in food allergy and that immune cells may also be involved. They also believe that specific food allergies can be measured and graded by skin and blood tests.

FOOD ALLERGY (Generalizations)

	FOOD	AIRBORNE
OCCURENCE	PERENNIAL	SEASONAL
SYMPTOMS	DIVERSE	LOCALIZED
ANTIBODY	IgG	IgE
REACTIONS	DELAYED	IMMEDIATE

THE TELLTALE SIGNS OF FOOD ALLERGY

Children with food allergies are easy to spot. They look tired and pale and have dark circles or "shiners" under their eyes. Their noses have a horizontal crease caused by wiping their noses with their hands – a gesture called the "nasal salute." These children miss a lot of school due to earaches or ear infections. They may also develop rashes, leg cramps (heretofore called "growing pains"), abdominal cramps, constipation and/or diarrhea and bedwetting. They may have difficulty concentrating on their schoolwork and tend to be withdrawn and irritable. The good news is that these symptoms often disappear when allergenic foods are eliminated. We have observed countless children in our medical practices who were labelled "hyperactive," "depressed," and "learning disabled," who improved on an allergen free diet.

In adults, food allergies have been accused of precipitating migraine headaches and irritable bowel syndrome as well as more obvious conditions like asthma and eczema. Up to 75% of migraine episodes have been attributed to food sensitivity. Prime suspects are the amine-containing foods which include aged cheeses, wine, beer and pickled foods like herring. In our experience, many other foods can cause the head to throb including milk products, chocolate, beef, wheat and citrus fruits. The "irritable bowel" or "spastic colon" are catch-all phrases which describe any nagging digestive problem, including gas, cramps, constipation and/or diarrhea for which there is no clear explanation. Vast numbers of patients are stamped with these vague diagnoses and are treated with antacids, stomach acid blockers, smooth muscle relaxants, and tranquilizers. In our experience, it is often much easier and less costly to pacify an irritable bowel by eliminating food allergens from the diet.

FOOD ALLERGIES ARE ADDICTIONS

We owe much of our knowledge about food allergy to Dr. Theron Randolph, a noted allergist who has spent most of his long and illustrious career elucidating the complex nature of food allergy and the broad spectrum of its symptoms and its treatment. This has been an arduous task. Dr. Randolph has stretched our comprehen-sion of food allergy well beyond the traditional framework. He theorized that food allergy was a process that obeys the laws of addic-tion and, therefore, contains concepts of food craving, masking, tolerance, and withdrawal.

Most patients never suspect food allergy as a cause of their problems. This is because 90% of food reactions are "masked" or hidden. Masking occurs when foods are eaten frequently as is the case with day to day dietary staples. For example, someone who is allergic to milk and drinks milk every day may have no more than a mild but ever present stuffy nose. This symptom is taken for granted. Milk allergy is not suspected. When milk products are removed from this person's diet for several days, the runny nose and postnasal drip become pronounced. This is a withdrawal response which mimics the mechanism of narcotic drug withdrawal. In essence, this is "kicking" a food allergy. Dr. Randolph has described other ways in which food allergy obeys the laws of addiction:

CRAVING: People crave the very foods to which they are most sensitive. It is revealing to ask a patient what foods he would sorely miss if they were removed from the diet. If that person immediately blurts out "Doctor, you can take anything out of my diet except my cheese and yogurt", you can reasonably suspect an underlying cow's milk allergy. It also follows from this concept, that the most common food allergies in any country are reflected by the rate at which those foods are consumed. In the United States, for example, the foods which top the allergy scale are cow's milk, corn, wheat, hen's eggs, and soy. Corn and soy are relative newcomers to this list. They have risen in allergenic prominence in the past twenty years due to their widespread inclusion in processed foods.

TOLERANCE: According to Dr. Randolph, the initial food allergy reaction is experienced as stimulation or a "high". After a varying period of time, the "high" may disappear and only return if more of that very food is consumed. The need to consume more and more of the addicting food to achieve the same "high" is called "tolerance".

WITHDRAWAL: If the allergenic food is not consumed in sufficient amounts to maintain tolerance, a withdrawal reaction may occur. This happens frequently overnight when ten to twelve hours pass without a food "fix" and one awakens with the early morning blues. Withdrawal symptoms mimic malaise and include fatigue, weakness, aches, and pains, and a general hungover feeling.

CHEMICAL HYPERSENSIVITY

Hypersensitivity to environmental chemicals is a growing public nightmare that afflicts an estimated 15% of the American public.[10] Patients with CFS often complain of a heightened sensitivity to environmental chemicals. These chemical offenders include fumes emanating from cosmetics, perfumes, smog, cigarette smoke, synthetic carpets, newsprint, copier machines, plywood, fabrics, vinyl, household cleaners, and other ordinary civilized chemicals. These chemicals saturate our daily, industrialized living environment. Patients with "environmental sensitivity" or "E.I." (Environmental Illness) are hypersensitive, even to minute exposures; these chemicals can produce a panoply of disabling symptoms. These symptoms must place E.I. high on the differential diagnosis of CFS.

As the twentieth century draws to a close, it leaves behind an environment contaminated with chemicals. This massive pollution is a sad remnant of the age of technology. It is a sobering and staggering realization that the United States annually generates over one hundred billion pounds of hazardous waste. This waste is dumped in landfills which contaminate our water supply with up to 700 foreign chemicals; to pick one glaring example, 20% of California's public water wells are contaminated! The agriculture business sprays over two billion pounds of pesticides on American crops every year. Ninety-nine percent of these chemicals never hit a single pest. The U.S. Environmental Protection Agency (EPA) estimates that most Americans store low levels of over 100 foreign chemicals in their bodies; many are known carcinogens.

Life forms can adapt to routine environmental insults. The human body degrades chemical toxins in the liver and excretes them in sweat and urine. Body fat stores residual chemicals in depots which we choose to call "The Biodump." These chemicals seep out of the body gradually, except when there is rapid weight loss, such as following a crash diet, during which the body may release a chemical avalanche. This modern chemical onslaught surpasses the routine which our bodies expect; this appears in some people to overwhelm their defenses, resulting in an increasing population reeling from environmentally-caused illnesses and even cancer. No prior generation has had to cope with the magnitude of this chemical overload.

In 1985, the Canadian government reported that environmental disease is a real and growing phenomenon and deserves detailed study. In 1987, the U.S. National Academy of Sciences held a workshop on "Health Risks from Exposure to Common Household Products in Allergic and Chemically Diseased Persons" which reinforced the urgent need for further studies. In late 1989, the State of New Jersey Department of Health published a comprehensive report on "Chemical Sensitivity," based on an exhaustive review of the literature and in-depth interviews with "E.I." patients and physicians who specialize in environmental medicine. This report stated at the outset that there is *"sufficient evidence to conclude that chemical sensitivity does exist as a serious health and environmental problem... and that chemical sensitivity is increasing and could become a large problem with significant economic consequences related to the disablement of productive members of society."*

What is the chemical hypersensitivity syndrome?(CHS)

The New Jersey report defines it systematically:

1. CHS is caused by chemical exposure, which may be acute and massive or prolonged and low grade.
2. Sensitivity develops to minute levels of the offending chemical which do not affect the average person.
3. Symptoms develop due to chemical exposure which are localized at first to a specific body part.
4. As the exposure continues, sensitivity develops to a range of environmental substances which may be chemically unrelated to the original incitant. This is called "Multi-Chemical Sensitivity" (MCS).
5. The "spreading" phenomenon occurs as symptoms spread to other body parts. At this stage, malaise, lethargy and generalized aches and pains accompany other localized complaints.

The official New Jersey report defines chemical hypersensitivity as a disease process which occurs in stages.

We appreciate this report but feel that one step is missing. That step is called "Susceptibility." Many people can experience the same degree of chemical exposure but only some develop environmental illness. Many theories abound as to the underlying causes of such host susceptibility, among them:

1. Immune dysregulation which may be an inherited genetic defect or due to the immune scrambling effects of a chronic infection. This possiblity we believe is the link to CFS. The viruses implicated in CFS disrupt the immune response and may lay the groundwork for chemical sensitivity. As we have stated, chemical sensitivity is common among CFS patients but its presence has been largely ignored in most medical publications.
2. Incapacity of the liver to detoxify chemicals possibly due to a heavy chemical load. This liver insufficiency may be crudely measured by urine levels of glucaric and mercapturic acids.
3. Adrenal gland insufficiency due to stress which is known to cause hypersensitivity to sound and light. Why not to smells?

THE PROGRESSION OF MULTI-CHEMICAL SENSITIVITY

1. EXPOSURE
2. SUSCEPTIBILITY
3. SENSITIVITY
4. LOCALIZED SYMPTOMS
5. MULTICHEMICAL SENSITIVITY
6. SPREADING SYMPTOMS

The saga of Larry K. illustrates the progression of Multi-Chemical Sensitivity. Notice particularly as you read his story how easily one could mistake his case for CFS. Indeed, this could be a true CFS if we could diagnose it with certainty.

In 1988, Larry was earning a six figure income as a computer consultant for a large corporation. He had toiled long and demanding hours for ten years in a "tight building" with no open windows in the smoggy environs of Silicon Valley. In the winter of 1986, Larry recalls coming down "with a bad flu." He simply never recovered. At first, he complained of recurrent flu-like symptoms like malaise, swollen glands and a low grade sore throat. His lethargy and overall malaise persisted and got worse. He developed a fullblown CFS picture. But, there was another disabling aspect to his story. Three months after he caught the flu, Larry noticed that he became sick whenever he entered his workplace. *"A room full of computers gave me an instant headache. I couldn't think straight. After a while, I could actually detect the smell of a single computer operating in a large room."* Within a few months, Larry "became supersensitive to the whole world." He could detect the smells of cosmetics and colognes emanating from other rooms. Perfumes, gas fumes, cigarette smoke and smog all made him feel sick. His symptoms spread to his "whole body". *"I just felt awful. Obviously, I couldn't work anymore."*

Larry is now forced to subsist on disability. He has adopted a spartan approach to the outside world. He avoids department stores, movie theaters, supermarkets and freeways. He stays indoors on smoggy days and has an air filter running all the time. He stripped his indoor environment of chemical pollutants like gas heating, synthetic carpeting, particle board and vinyl furniture. He shuns polyester clothing and scented toiletries. Larry is chemically disabled.

The outlook for patients like Larry is guarded. Generally, rehabilitation is a slow and gradual process. It may take months or even years of living in a relatively chemical free environment to give the body a chance to heal. It is also important to reduce overall stress and to treat chronic and hidden infections including yeast and parasites. Many patients derive some benefit by taking anti-oxidant vitamin supplements. The theory here is that petrochemicals form free radicals inside our body which can damage the liver and immune system and cause chemical sensitivity. Anti-oxidants counter these free radicals.

The chemical hypersensitivity syndrome is not well accepted in medical circles, and has been recently criticized for its lack of double-blind tests to establish it. We expect the controversy to persist about its validity because such cases are extremely complicated and demand a great deal of skill and knowledge by the licensed health care practitioner. In most cases, E.I. patients have been relegated to the psychiatric doghouse. They are said to be suffering from depression, paranoia, hysterical conversion disorders, and borderline personality traits. Indeed, it would not surprise us that many, if not most, E.I. patients have some psychiatric problems as a result of their illness. The extreme stress of a chemical disability in some patients is enough to provoke mental illness. The medical profession has to face up to the fact that psychiatric problems can accompany viral fatigue syndromes and environmental illness without negating the existence of these conditions.

E.I. could be the link between the immune system and CFS. E.I. could be a cause or an effect of CFS—or, of course, it could be the vicious cycle leading to both in some patients.

References

1. Goldstein, J.A. Personal communication, 1990.
2. Goldstein, J.A. *Chronic Fatigue Syndrome: The Struggle For Health.* Chronic Fatigue Institute, Beverly Hills, CA, 1990.
3. Selye, H. *Stress Without Distress.* Harper and Row, New York, 1974.
4. Patterson, C.C., H.Shirahata, and J.E. Ericson. Lead in Ancient Roman Bones and Its Relevance to Historical Developments of Social Problems With Lead. In: *The Science of the Total Environment,* Elsevier Science., Amsterdam, 61; 167-200, 1987.
5. Environmental Protection Agency of U.S.: *Reducing Lead in Drinking Water: A Benefit Analysis.* Dec. 1986.
6. American College of Advancement in Medicine (ACAM): Laguna Hills, CA, Phone 714-583-7666.
7. Schroeder, Henry A. *The Trace Elements and Man,* The Devin-Adair Company, Old Greenwich, Connecticut, 1973.
8. Huggins, H. *It's All In Your Head.* Life Sciences Press, Tacoma, WA, 1989.
9. Werbach, M. *Nutritional Influences on Disease.* Third Line Press, Encino, CA., 1988.
10. Estimate -National Academy of Science. 1987.

CHAPTER 8

THE IMMUNE SYSTEM

The immune system is the most dynamic system in the body. Its cells reproduce at a phenomenal rate.

"Immunity" means freedom. From its Latin roots, the word immunity actually means freedom from taxation. In our bodies, the immune system protects us from being taxed by the relentless pursuit of microbial pathogens. We coexist with a vast population of microscopic armies consisting of viruses, bacteria, yeast and parasites who are literally trying to feed off us. The immune system is our major defense against this constant siege. For this reason we will dedicate an entire chapter to this technical and demanding specialty in medicine.

To combat a never ending hoard of enemies, the immune system must be dynamic and ever vigilant. In fact, the immune system is the most dynamic system in the body. Its cells reproduce at a phenomenal rate equated only by the cells of the brain in sheer numbers. The immune system is highly intricate and consists of both cells providing "cellular immunity" and secreted substances providing "humoral immunity." There is a complex and sensitive interplay between immune cells and the chemical mediators they secrete.

The most primitive of the cell types are called "phagocytes." When seen under the microscope, these cells contain many granules and are also called "granulocytes." These are the scavengers of the immune system. They wander through the blood stream and extravascular spaces searching for microbes on the loose. They are capable of ingesting and destroying microbes and cell debris. A particular type of scavenger cell called the "macrophage" has an even more glorious role. It not only consumes and destroys foreign substances but also has the capability of processing these agents for presentation to the "higher" and newer part of the immune system—governed by cells called "lymphocytes."

The macrophages use their radar to detect and announce the presence of an invader. Macrophages can ingest an entire microbe or tumor cell, remove its identifying label and wear it on its own outer membrane. This process alerts the lymphocytes to scan the label to detect if it is friend or foe. Macrophages also secrete a small protein called "IL-1" (interleukin-1) which activates lymphocytes to respond to the attack. Activated lymphocytes are the most highly specific cells of the immune system. They secrete another small protein or "peptide" called "IL-2" (interleukin-2), which rapidly summons a diverse brigade of immune cells to join the fight. IL-2 amplifies every aspect of the immune attack. It increases the number of all activated lymphocytes which include "T cells" and "B cells" All lymphocytes originate in the bone marrow. One class of lymphocytes migrate to the thymus gland located in the upper chest where they mature into "T" (for Thymus) cells. The T cells seem to orchestrate the entire immune response. There are four main types of T cells:

1. T Helpers which amplify (up regulate)
2. T Suppressors which reduce (down regulate)
3. T Cytotoxic cells which can directly attack target invader cells
4. Null cells which contain Killer or "K" cells and Natural Killer or "NK" cells both of which can target cells laden with virus or malignancy.

IL-2 also stimulates the other major type of lymphocyte called "B cells." The "B cells" mature into "plasma cells" and "memory cells." Plasma cells are really the munitions factory of the immune army. These cells produce antibodies which are proteins consisting of two sets of paired chains that function like guided missiles. They are made to conform exactly and bond to a small portion of the invader called the "epitope." They immobilize and neutralize the attack. The memory cells retain the specific label of the epitope for the rest of one's life and can quickly summon an antibody response if the invader reappears.

The immune system is equipped with an exquisite memory. Antibodies are also called immunoglobulins or "Ig." The antibodies that protect us from viruses, bacteria and yeast are types "G" and "M" ("IgM" and "IgG").

IgM is the first antibody that is mobilized following an assault by a new pathogen. This is called the "primary immune response" and takes a few weeks for its level to peak. Subsequently, the "secondary immune response" occurs. IgG levels rise slowly and predominate thereafter. There are 4 sub-classes of IgG called appropriately IgG1, 2, 3, or 4. IgG types 1 and 3 protect us from viruses and are most relevant to our discussion of CFS. There is also another class of antibody that is present in body secretions and which acts as a first line defense against infections. It is called secretory IgA. It is present in saliva (where it may be conveniently measured by a laboratory) and in the fluids secreted by the gastro-intestinal and genito-urinary tracts. Babies do not manufacture IgA until six months of age and must depend on the IgA present in human breast milk for this first line defense

IgG is 75% of all antibodies
IgA 15%
IgM 10%
IgE 0.005% or infinitesimal

MORE AMMUNITION

There is another part of the humoral immune system called "complement." These are enzymatic proteins, about twenty in all, which activate each other in a serial fashion, step by step, and have powerful immune effects along the way. These enzymes are present to "complement" the whole process of phagocytosis by encouraging "chemotaxis" which is the speedy movement of the scavenger cells. It also encourages the binding of the phagocyte to its prey and the release of the granules so deadly to the prey. "Complement" can also lyse a target cell directly.

SPECIFIC and NON SPECIFIC IMMUNE CELLS

SPECIFIC	NON SPECIFIC
NEW IMMUNE CELLS	PRIMITIVE IMMUNE CELLS
T AND B LYMPHOCYTES	GRANULOCYTES
'K' or KILLER CELLS	PMN CELLS
ANTIBODIES	EOSINOPHILES, BASOPHILS
	MACROPHAGES
	"NK" or NATURAL KILLER CELLS

CYTOKINES

One of the exciting new topics in immunology is the discovery of "cytokines." These are small protein substances, secreted by macrophages and lymphocytes that act like immune messengers. Cytokines communicate messages between immune cells and act to modulate the immune response. There may be hundreds of these messengers of which IL-1 and IL-2 are prime examples. Interferons are also types of cytokines which are front line inhibitors of viral reproduction.

IMMUNE REGULATION

The immune system has such a rapid turnover of cells, it is exquisitely vulnerable to changes thrust upon it by external circumstances. The immune response may be modulated by the aging process, stress, diet, vitamin and mineral supplements, a variety of medications, exercise and emotions.

Think of the immune system as a vast military service fighting a never ending war! As an example, the United States military consists of a central executive command called the Pentagon. Beneath it lie military divisions: the Army, Navy and Air Force, each of which consists of commissioned officers of various rank and the non-commissioned troops below them. The military requires vehicles like planes, trucks, tanks, weapons, ammunition, and a spy service capable of intercepting, deciphering and remembering enemy messages. The immune system is analagous to this military model.

PENTAGON	THYMUS GLAND	
MILITARY INSTALLATIONS	BONE MARROW	LYMPH NODES
MILITARY DIVISIONS	PHAGOCYTES	LYMPHOCYTES
OFFICERS	NK CELLS	NK CELLS T & B CELLS
INFANTRY	MACROPHAGES PMNs, EOSINOPHILS	
WEAPONS & AMMUNITION	LYSOSOMAL GRANULES	ANTIBODIES
COMMUNICATIONS		CYTOKINES

The NK or "natural killer cell" is placed under both "PHAGOCYTE" and "LYMPHOCYTE" because it shares characteristics of both cells. It looks like a large lymphocyte and possesses excellent surveillance capabilities to detect tumor and virus laden cells. However, it behaves like a phagocyte because it is nonspecific in action and destroys cells by secreting lysosomal granules. It is noteworthy that a major subset of NK Cells is reduced or missing in CFS patients. The immune system has an extremely rapid turnover in its infantry cells, the phagocytes. These cells reproduce at the astonishing rate of one hundred billion cells for each cell type each day to replace the one hundred billion cells that have expired. That leaves precious little time for basic training! Once produced, these cells have a lifespan of about four days. Comparing that to our military would mean replacing the entire infantry every four days! That is but one reason why our immune system is the most dynamic organ system in the body and should be regarded with a sense of awe and appreciation.

How can such a system regulate itself? It has many divisions and a phenomenal rate of turnover of its components. Consider the problem of fine tuning such a system. Remember, also, that the body's military is always at war. It is constantly under attack. There are always invaders trespassing through our portals of entry: the mouth, nose, skin, genitals and urinary tract.

The immune system requires exquisite care. One must supply it with the right quality of food, air and water. Contaminants and deficiencies cause mishaps. Malnutrition damages the immune system more than any other organ system in the body! Insults from a wide variety of medications, recreational drugs, and alcohol compound the damage. Chronic pain and emotional problems, including anxiety, depression and relentless worry also exact their toll on this powerful but delicate system.

A SIMPLE SCHEME OF IMMUNE REGULATION

The Thymus: The thymus secretes 5 hormones called "thymosins." These are small proteins with the capacity to up- and down-regulate the proliferation and maturation of immune cells. Via these hormones, the thymus orchestrates the entire immune show. The thymus does not act independently. It interacts with a variety of hormones and the nervous system. The hypothalamus, that portion of the brain which controls our emotions and vegetative needs, has been shown to exert sensitive control over the thymus gland. This may explain the negative effects of emotional upsets and sleep deprivation.

Cytokines: Cytokines are chemical messengers composed of small protein units called peptides that are made by lymphocytes and macrophages. There may be hundreds of these messengers which modulate the immune response and inflammation. It will probably take years to clarify the vast role that cytokines play in human immunity.

Important Cytokines: Interleukin 1 (IL-1 "Interleukin" means "between white blood cells." IL-1 is made by macrophages and activates T Cells to respond to a specific antigen. Interleukin 2 (IL-2): IL-2 is subsequently generated by the activated T Helper Cell. It, in turn, activates all the other "officer cells" including other T Helpers, Killers, Natural Killers and B cells.

These cytokines not only boost the immune response, they also may make us feel sick. For instance, IL-1 causes us to have a fever. IL-2 can cause all the symptoms that we typically associate with having a flu-like malaise and body aches. Is it not interesting that our own immune response can make us feel sick! In some ways, the immune system resembles the nervous system. It makes us experience malaise to let us know that we are sick in order to rest and maximize our immune defences. Malaise could be called the equivalent of metabolic pain. Just as pain warns about something structurally wrong with an organ, malaise says there is something metabolically wrong.

IMMUNE DYSREGULATION

There are two types of immune deficiencies: Primary or inherited and Secondary or acquired. Inherited immunodeficiencies are relatively rare and occur mostly in children. Acquired immune difficiency is common. We are now faced with a scourge of acquired immune diseases of which AIDS is only one. What is it about the late twentieth century that seems to be scrambling the immune response? Several theories arise:

THE LAST STRAW THEORY

This theory states that the immune system seems to collapse under the weight of collective environmental abuses. Remember that the immune system is sensitive to environmental insults:

Exposure to infections in poor, overcrowded neighborhoods
Pollutants and toxins in food, air and water
Malnutrition
Stress
Recreational drugs
Prescription drugs including tranquilizers and sleeping pills.

THE COMMON ENDPOINT THEORY

This theory states that many different microbes can dysregulate immunity producing the entire symptom complex that we call CFS. Think about the common cold. Hundreds of viruses can cause it, yet they all feel the same to the victim. For several years, it was thought that any one of a number of Herpes viruses could independently cause CFS. This outlook is losing favor.

THE SINGLE AGENT THEORY

A specific agent, thought to be a virus, initiates an immune dysregulation. A mixed infection follows. All the varied symptoms that occur are lumped together under the heading "Chronic Fatigue Syndrome". The latest candidate for this mysterious single agent is a retrovirus.

A COMBINATION THEORY

We favor a combination of these three theories into the following scheme:

SETTING THE STAGE

A gradual immune decline occurs due to repeated abuse of the sensitive immune apparatus by years of consuming a typical Western high calorie, high fat diet, use of birth control pills and tranquilizers, exposure to environmental toxins like lead, mercury, cadmium, pesticides in fruits and vegetables and insecticides. Chronic stress seems also to play a key role in "setting the stage." But sudden massive stress like a death in the family, a divorce or loss of a job, is often the final blow that precipitates a long-term bout of CFS.

ENTER THE MYSTERIOUS SINGLE AGENT

This probable retrovirus enters the scene and causes a profound immune dysregulation. The immune system goes out of synch. In some ways, it is "up regulated" by overproducing unneeded antibodies that may cause allergies or auto immune diseases. In other ways, it is "down regulated" by underproducing vital virus-fighting antibodies and Natural Killer Cells.

THE MIXED INFECTION SYNDROME

When key IgG antibodies are low and NK Cells are missing, the Herpes family of viruses can flourish along with yeasts and parasites. The hapless immune system must take on too many contenders at once which further depletes its reserves. Is it any wonder that, at this stage, people become totally exhausted and hurt all over? Obviously, we cannot yet treat Factor 2, the single agent, because its identity is still a mystery. But, we can intervene with Factors One and Three by reducing environmental factors that disrupt the immune response and eradicating the mixed infections that are present. This combined and integrative approach is the major reason for our success. And yet, these Factors are often overlooked.

IMMUNE PROBLEMS ASSOCIATED WITH CFS

DOWN REGULATION:

LOW ANTIBODY LEVELS. Low IgG1, Low Secretory IgA
LOW CELL MEDIATED IMMUNITY - as measured by skin tests
LOW NATURAL KILLER CELLS
LOW CYTOKINES - Gamma Interferon, IL-1 and TNF (Tumor necrosis factor) Alpha.

UP REGULATION:

HIGH CYTOKINES - High Interleukin 2, High TGF - Beta
Elevated T Helper/ Suppressor Ratios.
Elevated numbers of B Cells.
Elevated Circulating Immune Complexes by Rajii analysis in about 70%.
High Plasma Histamine in about 75%. (This may contribute to nasal congestion, acid stomach, itching and diarrhea) Elevated levels of auto antibodies - ANA, Thyroid Antibodies.

One half of all CFS patients have high levels of interleukin 2 (Cheney and Bell, *Ann. Int. Med.*, 1989). On the average, these levels are eleven times higher than in the normal population! More IL-2 is all it takes to up regulate the entire immune response.

CHAPTER 9

NUTRITION AND IMMUNITY

This is a surprise. Serum levels of antibodies usually remain normal or may even be increased in certain kinds of malnutrition.

The information explosion in immunology during the past decade has included a surge of interest in the varied roles that diet and individual nutrients play in the immune response. The food-immunity connection has been explored for over a century. A good deal of the research has narrowly focused on the ill effects of severe protein and calorie malnutrition on infectious diseases in impoverished third world countries. This condition is called PEM (Protein Energy Malnutrition) and is the most frequent cause of acquired immunodeficiency in the world! Its victims are primarily children, pregnant women, and the elderly. In the mid-nineteen eighties, the world was witness to the ravages of famine in Ethiopia and the spectre of hoards of dying children. These children suffered from a lack of adequate protein and the vitamins and minerals that support protein synthesis. These co-factors include Vitamin B6, folic acid and zinc. But PEM is not limited to poor countries like Ethiopia! The western world is also afflicted. Until about two decades ago, little had been done to clarify the shocking extent of malnutrition and immunoincompetence in the United States and other affluent countries.

OVER and UNDER NUTRITION

As the saying goes, the western world is "overfed but undernourished." The sad facts about "over and under nutrition" in America were dramatized by the United States Senate Select Sub-Committee meetings on Nutrition held in 1978. This booklet became one of the most requested government publications in U.S. history. It was the first time that the United States government had publicly condemned the American diet.

The Senate report told us that the average American consumed an "empty calorie" diet consisting of over 40% of its calories as fat and 20% of its calories as refined sugar. The diet lacked natural fiber and exceeded twenty times the human requirement for salt, plus ten pounds of unnatural chemical food additives per person each year. Now, more than a decade has passed since the Senate nutrition report stirred up a national clamor. In the mid-nineteen eighties, the American Heart Association joined the campaign for less fat and more fiber. Poultry and fish began to replace steak and chops on the American plate. Bran consumption soared as labels on bread, muffins and cold cereals bragged about their fiber content. In spite of these promising developments, malnutrition still abounds in the land of plenty. Broad based surveys of the American diet confirm a continuing reliance on high fat, empty calorie foods. Marginal malnutrition is commonplace! Studies find, for example, women of college age to be lacking in iron, vitamin E, and B complex; the elderly typically lack zinc which is so vital to proper immune function. The United States Department of Agriculture estimates chromium to be low in ninety percent of the U.S. population. Even athletes suffer great risk of mineral deficiencies which include zinc, copper, magnesium and chromium. If seemingly healthy young women and athletes develop nutrient deficiencies, imagine how old age and chronic disease can compound the risk.

In the United States, studies reveal significant malnutrition in over 15% of patients entering acute care hospitals. This state of marginal malnutrition stems from poor appetite and malabsorption. The stress of surgery and infection make matters worse and plunges the patient into negative protein balance.

Now back to CFS. What does PEM do to immunity?

Protein-Energy Malnutrition (PEM) can devastate the immune response:

1. The thymus gland shrinks in size. Thymosin hormone levels drop.
2. There is a marked reduction in the number of mature circulating T Cells.
3. T Cells show a sluggish response to challenge by bacteria or viruses. IL-2 levels drop precipitously as the immune response falters.
4. T Helper Cells fall faster than the T Suppressors, thereby reducing the Helper/Suppressor ratio to very low levels.

5. Skin tests for cell mediated immunity may not swell as they should, even with agents that are common and with which the subjects have been previously vaccinated—like tetanus and diphtheria.
6. This may be a surprise. Serum levels of most antibodies usually remain normal or may even be increased. The paradox is that these antibodies may not work. This action of quantity without quality means that antibody levels are not a good measure of immunocompetence in malnutrition.
7. In contrast, secretory IgA antibodies do decline. Remember that these antibodies do not only circulate in the bloodstream but are a first line of local defense against infection in our nose, lungs, intestines and bladder.
8. The number of circulating phagocytes may be normal. In fact, these "PacMan" cells may have normal mobility and can engulf bacteria with their usual gusto. However, they have difficulty destroying what they swallow.

In summary, PEM results in depression of cell-mediated immunity. Antibodies are normal in number, but may not work. Phagocytes cannot destroy their ingested prey. When these factors prevail, CFS may invade and pervade.

INDIVIDUAL NUTRIENTS and IMMUNITY

NUTRIENTS THAT HELP MAKE PROTEINS

ZINC and VITAMIN B-6

If we were forced to choose the most important nutrient for immunity, it would be zinc. Zinc is a potent immunostimulant; we know of no other nutrient which can stimulate lymphocytes to reproduce when incubated with them in a test tube. This biological property is called a "mitogen effect." Zinc deficiency often accompanies PEM and seems the major cause of the weak immunity of severe malnutrition. In retrospect, it might have been wise to send zinc supplements to Ethiopia during the famine.

Zinc is a mineral co-factor in over eighty enzyme reactions in the human body. Zinc acts as a paramount growth factor; it is essential to the health of the growing fetus and small child. Cells that reproduce quickly are in desperate need of a steady supply of zinc. It is no wonder then that zinc deficiency causes stunted growth, poor sexual development, skin lesions, hair loss, and a susceptibility to infection. The immune damage that occurs appears indistinguishable from that seen in PEM. PEM and zinc deficiency intertwine endlessly with CFS in this ongoing drama.

Does zinc deficiency occur in America? Not only does it occur, it is commonplace—for many reasons: the average American diet, at best, manages to be borderline in zinc content. Zinc uptake can be reduced by cadmium, mercury, and excessive levels of copper, since they all share the same protein carrier known as metallothionien. Obesity is associated with low blood levels of zinc. Diuretics, used in the treatment of high blood pressure, fluid retention, and premenstrual tension, increase zinc excretion in the urine. Alcohol, itself a marvelous diuretic, also depletes zinc stores. Aging doesn't help; the body's zinc levels tend to diminish with age, as does the immune response. As we become elderly, we become more susceptible to auto-immune diseases, infections, and cancer.

If zinc is such a potent immunostimulant, can zinc supplements restore the immune response in elderly people? The answer is a resounding and heartening "Yes!" Research has shown that a thirty milligram tablet of zinc taken each day for one month is sufficient to restore the mitogen response of lymphocytes in elderly people. A new form of liquid zinc can act quickly as a supplement to increase zinc status. Too much zinc, however, can be a hindrance. Excessive zinc in the range of 120 mg. or more per day can raise blood cholesterol and paralyze the phagocyte cells. In contrast, zinc deficiency causes macrophages to exhibit peak scavenger ability.

Pyridoxine (vitamin B-6) and zinc are both necessary for the synthesis of protein and seem to potentiate each other's effects on the immune system. Vitamin B-6 deficiency is more damaging to immune function than a deficiency of any other B vitamin. Deficiency of B-6 results in a loss of cell mediated immunity. The size and weight of the thymus decreases, and the total lymphocyte count diminishes; this usually does not occur with an isolated zinc deficiency. Vitamin B-6 deficiencies are common in women of child-bearing age. The female hormones, estrogen and progesterone, tend to consume vitamin B6 during their metabolism in the liver. Women who have had multiple pregnancies or long-term use of birth control pills are at special risk of developing a vitamin B-6 deficiency. Premenstrual tension has been attributed to a pyridoxine deficiency. It is noteworthy that the typical profile of a CFS patient is that of a stressed out professional woman in her child-bearing years.

ANTI-OXIDANTS

We need to breathe in order to obtain oxygen. This vital gas is utilized to "burn" carbohydrates and fat within our cells to produce energy. This process is called "oxidation" and is absolutely necessary to sustain human life. However, the process of oxidation is a double edged sword. It can also pose serious risks. The byproducts of oxidation are very short lived chemicals called "free radicals." An excess of free radicals has been shown to damage cell membranes and to attack the DNA in our genes causing mutations and even cancer. Other factors besides oxygen form free radicals. Other major sources include the unsaturated fatty acids found in vegetable oils. When used in frying, these hot oils form "epoxides" which are dangerous free radicals. Frying a steak can cause free radical epoxides to form from cholesterol. The cholesterol free radical can attack the walls of our arteries and cause heart disease. Ultraviolet rays from the sun and from tanning salons are another major source of free radicals. It is common knowledge that these free radicals cause skin cancer. The level of free radicals in our cells or in the bloodstream must be kept under strict control. How are we protected against these "radical" marauders? This vital role is performed by substances called "anti-oxidants", which are certain vitamins, minerals, and enzymes that can defuse or neutralize free radicals. They are aptly described as "free radical scavengers."

Anti-oxidants have attracted tremendous scientific attention and fascination over the past decade. There is a wealth of data to suggest that anti-oxidants can protect us against chronic degenerative diseases like heart disease, arthritis, and cancer—and may well promote longevity. They are also gaining an excellent reputation as immune stimulants. Generally, anti-oxidants stimulate the activity of phagocytes, the "Pac Men" of the immune system. These cells generate a massive amount of free radicals for a good purpose: to destroy the bacteria and yeast cells that they ingest. But what happens when phagocytes generate excess free radicals—because of lack of anti-oxidants? The sad truth is that a deficiency of anti-oxidants can cause these scavenger cells to leak free radicals. This constitutes an immune backfire, resulting in inflammation—swelling, pain, fever and malaise. What are the anti-oxidants? For the most part, they are nutrients that are present in any well balanced multi-vitamin and mineral supplement: vitamin C, vitamin E, beta-carotene, selenium and zinc. One relative newcomer to the anti-oxidant armamentarium in the last decade is Co-enzyme Q-10 or Co Q-10.

VITAMIN C

Linus Pauling is an eminent scientist and double Nobel laureate who is best known to the general public for his outspoken support of the health benefits of vitamin C. His book *Vitamin C, the Common Cold and the Flu,* has stirred a spirited controversy about the effects of vitamin C upon the immune response. During the past decade, many revealing studies on this relationship have been performed. It is unfortunate that few of these studies has employed the megadose of ten grams per day of vitamin C as recommended by Dr. Pauling. In fact, most studies utilized doses below one gram per day. However, at the relatively low doses of vitamin C that have been employed, the results have in most cases been described as generally modest but definite. Most authors agree that vitamin C supplementation results in a reduction in the severity and duration of the common cold. The best effects occur when vitamin C is administered at the earliest signs of illness.

Vitamin C works by pressing on the "gas pedal" of all phagocyte cells. Macrophages and neutrophils contain high amounts of vitamin C which accelerates the random motion of these scavengers to move much faster in all directions. This is of obvious benefit when chasing elusive microbes. For example, a 1980 study published in the *American Journal of Clinical Nutrition* investigated the effects of increasing doses of vitamin C upon the speed of neutrophils. In a three week study, human volunteers were given one gram of vitamin C per day the first week followed by two grams per day during the second week and three grams per day during the third week. Following each week, the speed of their neutrophils was measured. The results were striking. Two grams of vitamin C per day sparked these neutrophils to move three to four times faster than their original speed.[1] Lymphocytes also need vitamin C desperately. Viruses rapidly deplete lymphocytes of vitamin C. This may help to explain Dr. Pauling's insistence on megadoses of ascorbate in the treatment of serious viral infections like CFS. Similar findings were recently published in the *Clinical Guide to the Use of Vitamin C,* which cites the results of the world's foremost clinical practitioner of the use of vitamin C, the late Dr. Frederick R. Klenner. High doses of vitamin C have been shown to stimulate lymphocyte "transformation" which is their ability to reproduce and mature.[2] Vitamin C has one more important immune function. It increases the release of interferon, a major defense against virus attack. Again we see the nutrient-CFS connection.

ENZYME Q-10 (Co Q-10)

Coenzyme Q-10 is another nutrient supplement that made its way to the western world from Japan. The Japanese have done extensive research on Co Q-10 for over thirty years and regard it highly enough to recommend an average daily intake of 20 mg. per day. Co Q-10 is essential for life. Even a 25% body deficiency may result in serious illness. Rapid oxidation of sugar and fat for energy requires Co Q10. Therefore, cells with a rapid metabolism and a high demand for oxygen would have the most critical need for Co Q-10 and would be most at risk in the event of a Co Q-10 deficiency. These cells belong to the skeletal muscles, the heart, the brain, and the immune system.

Research conducted, both in Japan and at the University of Texas, has confirmed that a chronic Co Q-10 deficiency is a risk factor for:

A. Congestive heart failure
B. Cardiac arrythmia
C. High blood pressure
D. Muscular weakness and lethargy
E. Impaired cellular and humoral immunity (obviously important in CFS)
F. Obesity
G. Gum disease

It is especially pertinent to CFS patients that during virus infections, Co Q-10 levels in white blood cells fall precipitously. In combatting these infections, the immune cells undergo rapid turn-over which drains many nutrients, in particular, Co Q-10.

Furthermore, deficiencies of Co Q-10 are common for other reasons:

1. The highest content of Co Q-10 is found in organ meats—especially heart muscle. How many of us savor kidney or heart meat or for that matter, even liver?
2. Vegetables and grains contain Co Q-1 through Q-9 which are inactive in the human body. It takes a healthy liver to convert all the other Co Qs to Co Q-10. Much valuable Co Q is lost along the way. We find that many patients do not consume a great enough percentage of their diet in these most healthful foods.
3. The blood level of Co Q-10 diminishes inexorably with age. Like wrinkles, it just seems to happen. This deficiency may contribute to the creeping obesity, immune failure, and heart disease that accompany aging.

It is not difficult to see why Co Q-10 seems to play an important role in CFS—deficiency of yet another natural metabolite which in turn contributes to the immune dysregulation which we see in CFS.

VITAMIN E, SELENIUM, and BETA-CAROTENE

Vitamin C is a water based anti-oxidant. It dissolves easily in water and protects the fluid compartments of our body against free radicals. However, the lipid parts of our body, which comprise all of our cell membranes and the vital components of our nervous system, (the brain, spinal cord, and peripheral nerves), are not soluble in water; what protects them? Fortunately, nature has provided lipid soluble anti-oxidants for just that vital purpose. Vitamin E, selenium and beta-carotene work in tandem to protect cell membranes from lipid peroxidation by free radicals. These anti-oxidants are also important immune boosters. For example, the addition of only moderate amounts of vitamin E to animal feed enhances the animal's antibody response. This effect has been noted in chickens, mice, and guinea pigs injected with virulent strains of bacteria and viruses. This immunostimulatory effect is magnified if vitamin E is administered together with selenium. Selenium has been shown to increase the killer capacity of phagocytes, whereas vitamin C works mostly by boosting the speed of these cells.

Beta-carotene is the yellow pigment present in such foods as sweet potatoes and leafy greens. It is unique in that it protects us from the damaging effects of a particularly noxious form of free-radical called "singlet oxygen." It has been suggested as vitally important in protecting the lungs and mouth from the cancer-producing effects of tobacco smoke. Certain carotenoids have also been shown to reduce the incidence of cervical cancer. We must, therefore, conclude that all these nutrients may play vital roles in CFS treatment and prevention.

VITAMIN A

Beta-carotene is really a precursor to vitamin A and is found in fruits and vegetables; it is called "provitamin A." Each unit of carotene is composed of two units of vitamin A. The carotene is broken down to form vitamin A by the liver and small intestines at a rate that is determined by the body's need for vitamin A. Therefore, even vegetarians can obtain their daily requirement for vitamin A. Only diabetics and people with a low thyroid condition have difficulty converting carotene to vitamin A. Similar to carotene, vitamin A is a fat soluble vitamin. However, unlike beta-carotene, vitamin A is not an anti oxidant. In fact, it is very vulnerable to free-radical attack.

NON-SPECIFIC RESISTANCE

The effects of vitamin A on the immune response are unique and fundamentally different from those of beta-carotene. Vitamin A, or "retinol," has been known for some time to enhance non-specific resistance to a wide variety of infectious organisms.

Vitamin A acts to preserve the integrity of the skin and mucous membrane linings throughout the body making it difficult for offensive agents to penetrate within. Vitamin A also lubricates the lining with tears, sweat, saliva and mucous and fortifies these secretions with "lysozyme" enzymes to destroy foreign proteins. Vitamin A deficiency in laboratory animals produces an immune disaster. The thymus shrinks and blood lymphocyte levels dwindle. The antibody response to infectious agents is reduced. In contrast, vitamin A supplementation directly enhances both cell-mediated and humoral immunity. What is particularly important for humans with CFS is that megadoses of vitamin A have been shown to prevent the immunosupression caused by extreme stress. An eye-opening study was performed in 1979, on three continents, to study the effects of the administration of 300,000 units of vitamin A a day on the immune response of people following extensive surgery. It is well known that surgery often suppresses the immune response profoundly for about a month. Of course, a healthy immune response is critical, after surgery, to prevent infections which have become all too common in hospital wards. In this experiment, the vitamin A treated group exhibited much heightened T cell activity whereas the control group, receiving no vitamin A, showed the classic signs of immunosupression. The authors concluded: "When compared with untreated patients after an operation, the results of these tests indicate that vitamin A is capable of blocking the depression of immune function associated with an operation and acting as an immunostimulant in man."[4]

IRON

Iron deficiency is probably the most common single nutrient deficiency in the world, afflicting vegetarians, menstruating women, malnourished children, and the elderly. Our bodies maintain a careful homeostasis of this critical mineral which carries oxygen to all our cells. Both iron deficiency and iron excess cause immune dysfunctions and increase the risk of infection. Iron deficiency impairs the killer capacity of phagocytes. Iron excess supplies iron to hungry bacteria and yeast cells which is vital for their replication. Our bodies take extra precautions to reduce the availability of iron when we are sick. Intestinal absorption of iron is reduced. White blood cells secrete a chemical that lowers the blood level of iron which is deployed to the liver until the infection has subsided. It may be dangerous to take iron supplements during the course of an infection. There is ample documentation in the medical literature about iron supplements increasing the hazards of sepsis in malnourished individuals.

OBESITY and IMMUNITY

Obesity is the most common nutritional disorder in industrialized countries. Obesity has a deleterious effect upon certain immune functions and tends to promote the incidence of infectious illness. Infection related mortality is also increased. These findings are supported by clinical and laboratory findings in humans and animals. A study of obese children and adults by Dr. Ranjit K. Chandra, a leading nutritional immunologist, showed that approximately one third of obese people had impairments in cell-mediated immunity and reduced killing capacity of neutrophils. What is the connection between obesity and low immunity? It may be malnutrition involving two key trace minerals—zinc and iron. Plasma zinc levels are low in the obese of all age groups. Low zinc could explain the reduction in cell mediated immunity. Low iron levels would impair the 'killer' capacity of phagocytes. Dr. Chandra reported that those obese subjects in his study who had weak scavenger abilities were the very persons with overt evidence of iron deficiency. It is good news that just one month of iron supplementation restored phagocytic functions to normal. There is no clear explanation for the low levels of zinc and iron in obese people. It does appear that supplementation with these two minerals may benefit the immune response.

DIETARY FAT and IMMUNITY

We have been warned repeatedly that high fat diets are a major risk factor for cardiovascular diseases and cancer. The American diet, which supplies over 40% of its total calories as fat, has been implicated as a cause of six of the ten leading chronic degenerative diseases.[3] It is becoming clear that high fat diets suppress immunity. It doesn't matter whether the fats are saturated or unsaturated! Vegetable oils may help to prevent heart disease, but excess amounts offend the immune response as much as prime rib. In laboratory animals, a high dietary intake of vegetable oils produces involution of the thymus gland and lymph glands with a concomitant decline in both cell mediated and humoral immunity. Macrophages and neutrophils have difficulty engulfing and destroying bacteria.

The more unsaturated the oil, the greater is its immunosupressant effect. The least unsaturated of the vegetable oils are olive, peanut and canola. Are these oils safer to use as far as immune function?

Presumably so, however, it is not really clear what dietary level of polyunsaturated fatty acids (PUFAs) is immunosuppressive in humans. We do know that the content of vegetable oils has increased markedly in the American diet during the twentieth century. Some researchers even think that PUFAs are a double edged sword, and can even cause rather than diminish heart disease in high doses. The *Journal of Cancer Research* carried an important paper which stated that "Diets high in PUFAs relative to saturated fat are both immunosupressive and promoters of tumorogenesis (cancer)."[4]

So, which should we decrease—hamburgers or salad oil? The evidence suggests that we cut down on both. Present evidence suggests that the optimal intake of dietary fat lies somewhere between 10 to 20 percent of total calories a day. Cutting down too much, however, can also endanger us. A deficiency of vital vegetable oils can also inhibit the immune response. Once again, moderation is the answer; once again a link between overall health and CFS.

VITAMIN D

The sunshine vitamin may put our immune system in the dark! An article published in 1984 in the journal *Science,* indicated that vitamin D suppressed the output of Interleukin 2 from normal human lymphocytes *in vitro.* This effect was directly related to the amount of vitamin D incubated with the white blood cells. Vitamin D is really a hormone! It is a steroid hormone similar in structure to cortisone and the female sex hormones. Steroid hormones as a class tend to reduce the immune response. Therefore, it should be no surprise that excess vitamin D may be an immune suppressant. How much vitamin D does it take to break the immune back? No one really knows. But, there is evidence that Americans may be getting overdosed with vitamin D from a combination of using vitamin D fortified milk products and multivitamins. There is no evidence, however, that too much sunlight exposure results in the synthesis of an excess of vitamin D.

TOXIC HEAVY METALS

In chapter 7, we outlined some of the health dangers posed by exposure to the heavy metals lead, cadmium and mercury. These toxic metals have all been shown to suppress immunity when tested in laboratory animals. All aspects of the immune response are squelched. Susceptibility to infection increases. Of course, the degree of immune impairment depends on the level of exposure. The risks to us are severalfold: these heavy metals are now omni-present in our contaminated environment in food, air and water. What we absorb, we keep! These metals are stored within our bodies and bio-accumulate with the passage of time. Cadmium that has accumulated in the body has a half life in human tissue of between 20 to 30 years. That means that if we get twice the amount of those heavy metals than our immune system can tolerate, we will take 20 years of natural excretion to be back to tolerable amounts. Therefore, we must take definate steps to discover and correct any excessive body burden of such toxic metals.

SUMMARY OUTLINE of NUTRITION and IMMUNITY

1. Up regulation of cell mediated and humoral immunity: Key nutrients: vitamin B-6, folic acid, vitamins A, C, E, zinc, and Co-enzyme Q-10. Any nutrient deficit can be damaging.
2. Down regulation of cell mediated immunity: Key Nutrients: polyunsaturated fatty acids, vitamin D
3. Stimulation of phagocyte functions: Key Nutrients: vitamin C, E, selenium, and iron.
4. Reduction of phagocyte functions: Key Toxins: Heavy metals—lead, mercury, cadmium (which are pure toxins). Zinc in high doses.

It is becoming clear that nutritional status plays a vital role in the immune response. The interaction between nutrition and immunity has an immense impact upon public health. These two burgeoning fields are uniting in a manner that will someday redefine the practice of medicine. In Chapter 10, we expand on our therapeutic approach to CFS.

REFERENCES

1. Anderson, R. *et al.* The Effects of Increasing Weekly Doses of ascorbate on certain cellular and humoral immune functions in normal volunteers. *Am J Clin Nutr.*, 1980: 33; 71-76.
2. Smith, L. *Clinical Guide to the Use of Vitmin C.* Life Sciences Press: Tacoma, 1991.
3. US Senate Select Committee Report, Parker House: Berkeley, 1977.
4. Vitale, J. and Broitman, S. Lipids and immune function. *Cancer Res.*, 1981: 41: 3706-3710.

CHAPTER 10

TREATMENTS

Our approach is to maintain an aggressive and sustained attack directed at each of the multiple causes of this complex disease.

The range of treatments for CFS stretches from zero to infinity. Unfortunately for many patients with CFS the conventional approach usually hangs near the zero end of our continuum; it is almost nihilistic. There seems to be a fatalistic *"You have to live with it"* attitude among most physicians. This attitude strongly pervaded CFS in its earliest years.

In recent years, the tendency toward treating CFS has been to recommend antidepressants, or the use of histamine-2-blockers, which for a minority of patients does provide some symptomatic relief of symptoms. At the other extreme of the spectrum of treatment, we see the shotgun barrage. Patients might try anything and everything from standard medicine to "crystal power." The old adage that the understanding of a disease is inversely proportional to the number of treatments, certainly applies here. Because there is no simple cure, there are many recommendations.

In essence, we take a broad approach. Depending on the patient, we make an intense and aggressive attack on the disease, or rarely we may decide to wait and see. Our tendency definitely leans toward the aggressive side. We use a range of modalities while explaining to the patient that no definite cure exists for this indefinite disease—unless we find that the patient actually has CF from a diagnosable condition. We consider this a possibility in every patient until we have exhausted diagnostic reasonableness.

Our basic principle of treating true CFS presently pivots on the immune system. As we have stated and restated, the immune system depends on nutrients for its vitality and stability. It also abhors toxins and environmental stimulants that interfere in its functioning and viability. In this treatment chapter, and given the knowledge you have gained about CF and CFS in the previous nine chapters, we will specify some basic dietary objectives and supplement regimes which we use to bolster inadequate immunological functioning, and review various drugs being used to combat this syndrome. Naturally we vary these programs broadly to accommodate the biochemical individuality of our patients. Nevertheless, there are basic principles and programs which apply widely to CFS victims.

SPECIFIC TREATMENTS

Devising a treatment program for CFS is a complex task laden with pitfalls. For one, a sizable portion of the medical community still continues to deny the very existence of CFS; it even poses the question: Is there really a disease to treat? By now, I hope you are convinced that CFS is indeed *for real*.

DRUG TREATMENTS

Of those doctors who believe that CFS exists, a good many approach its treatment with an attitude of resignation: "There is no treatment; you just have to live with it." These doctors may provide drugs for symptom relief like pain killers, tranquilizers, anti-depressants and sleeping pills. As helpful as these medicines may be, they do not lessen the body's total burden of infection nor do they mobilize the body's own protective forces.

To take a more aggressive step, the anti-herpes drug *acyclovir* was introduced as a direct thrust against alleged CFS viruses—EBV, CMV and Herpes type 6. Unfortunately, clinical trials of acyclovir have shown only tenuous positive effects. Much more success has been achieved by "histamine-2 blocking agents" like Tagamet®, Zantac®, Pepcid® and Axid®. These drugs are used in general medicine to block the production of stomach acid in the treatment of heartburn, hiatus hernia and duodenal ulcers. But, they have also earned a new role in the treatment of CFS by blocking histamine receptors on T cells and acting as overall T cell immunostimulants. They also increase energy and alertness in a number of CFS patients.

Another histamine blocker named *doxepin* (a standard anti-depressant) has been used successfully to reduce insomnia and to reverse deficits in slow wave sleep that is common in CFS and fibromyalgia. With improved sleep, doxepin relieves the pain of tense and tender muscle knots occurring at pressure points throughout the body.

These drugs have become the standard ammunition of conventional medicine in treating CFS.

While we respect and often use these drugs, we prefer to take a broad and open-minded approach to the treatment of Chronic Fatigue Syndrome. Our approach is to maintain an aggressive and sustained attack directed at each of the multiple causes of this complex disease. We employ a range of essential modalities. At the same time we are educating the patient that "no cure exists" for this debilitating disease. Sometimes the answer to CFS is easy if we find that the patient has CF from a single readily treatable condition. We consider this a possibility in every patient until we have exhausted our diagnostic discoveries and conjectures.

A WORKING MODEL of CFS and its TREATMENT

From current medical and scientific data combined with our own clinical experience, we have extrapolated a working model of various factors contributing to CFS. This model serves to expand the concept of what causes CFS into a broad framework of mixed infections and immune dysregulation while enlarging the range of treatments available, including oral and injectable drugs and nutrients.

This model begins with an examination of potential immune suppression caused by environmental and genetic factors. Next we evaluate the presence of a mixed infection syndrome resulting in immune dysregulation. This encompasses evaluating both up and down regulation. Up regulation causes auto-immunity. Down regulation paralyzes the immune response thereby setting the stage for a mysterious virus or "agent X" as we call it, to swoop down and precipitate full-blown Chronic Fatigue Syndrome.

Although this approach is based on a series of hypothetical assumptions, it provides a rationale for each plausible step in our treatment model.

FOUR STEPS TO BEAT THE FATIGUE EPIDEMIC

We believe that CFS is a mixture of maladies. Some components of this mix easily expose their identity during treatment. Others elude detection and therapy. Steps one and two of this program describe treatments of readily apparent mixed infections and allied medical conditions. Steps 3 and 4 focus on mysterious conditions that elude diagnosis—like occult virus infections and central nervous system failures.

STEP 1. TREAT MIXED INFECTIONS

A careful medical history, a physical examination and laboratory tests can diagnose single or mixed infections. Bacteria often cause a hidden sinusitis or urinary tract infection. Bacteria of a type called spirochetes can cause Lyme disease and syphilis. These conditions are infrequent but may need to be ruled out. Candida can over-colonize the bowel, genitals, and urinary tract. Parasites lurk in the dark confines of the digestive tract. These microbes may contribute to an overall malaise and can be eliminated with medication and/or herbs.

STEP 2. TREAT MIXED CONDITIONS

This step involves conditions other than infections which often co-exist with CFS. It includes anemia, airborne and food allergies, chemical hypersensitivity, heavy metal toxicity, thyroid and adrenal gland insufficiency and thyroiditis (See Chapter 7).

STEP 3. TREAT THE CORE CFS VIRUSES

A. Neutralize or directly inactivate the viruses.
B. Stimulate the immune response.

STEP 4. HEAL THE NERVOUS SYSTEM

A. Enhance energy.
B. Enhance mental alertness and cognition.
C. Alleviate depression, anxiety, insomnia and pain.

For each category in steps #3 and #4, specific medications and supplements listed below may facilitate treatment. We have mentioned many of these substances elsewhere in the book. We feel that this list can give impetus to practitioners who treat CFS. We do not have general protocols which would apply to specific groups of patients. All patients bring their biochemical and immune individuality to their doctor. We intend this list of therapeutic possibilities to educate physicians about the range of treatment options available. Each must be assessed according to the patient's needs and tolerances. Combined with the other modalities discussed in this chapter and throughout the book, these possible therapies may allow doctors to increase their effectiveness in confronting CFS by considering these remedies.

Since each patient is unique, we provide no dosage levels. Determining doses takes skill and experience.

INACTIVATE VIRUSES

Key: D (a prescription drug) H (an herbal)
N (a nutrient) B (a botanical medicine)

NAME		ACTION
Monolauric Acid	N	A twelve carbon fatty acid. Similar to medium chain fatty acids used to kill yeast. Gets into membranes, increases cell leakage. Reportedly successful in treating herpes.
Egg Lecithin	N	The AL 721 mixture. Increases membrane fluid leakage. Used experimentally in HIV infections and hepatitis.
Lysine	N	An amino acid. Significant history of treatment against herpes viruses. Interferes with viral replication.
Quercetin	N	Anti-viral, anti-tumor activity. One of the most potent bioflavinoids available.
St. John's Wort	H	Active ingredient is hypericin which inactivates retroviruses, *in vitro*.
Leptotania	H	General anti viral effect.
Adenosine	D	This nucleoside has been successful in treating herpes viruses (through I.M. phosphate injection). It may work by inactivating the virus, by stimulating immunity, and increasing levels of cyclic AMP which increases energy.
Cysteine	N	Enhances lysine's effect on suppressing herpes virus.

STIMULATE IMMUNITY

NAME		ACTION
Zinc	N	Stimulates cellular and humoral immunity. The only known nutrient mitogen. Directly inhibits rhino-viruses (i.e. the "common cold").
Vitamin B-6	N	Stimulates antibody response
Vitamin A	N	Increases non-specific immunity. Increases maturation of T cells. Increases secretory IgA.
Antioxidants	N	(vitamins C, E, beta-carotene, and selenium) Stimulate macrophages, neutrophils and natural killer cells.

NAME		ACTION
Dimethyl Glycine	N	Stimulates cellular immunity.
Iron	N	Stimulates neutrophils, macrophages.
Coenzyme Q-10	N	Stimulates cellular immunity.
Echinacea	H	Stimulates cellular immunity, interferon.
Astragalus	H	Stimulates cellular immunity.
DHEA		Stimulates cellular immunity.
Shiitake Mushroom	N	(Lentinan fraction) Interferon induction tumor regression. *Only* effective by injection.
Garlic	N	Rich in anti-oxidants. Shown to be an NK cell stimulant.
Doxepin	D	Anti-depressant and potent H1 and H2 receptor antihistamine. In minute doses, it stimulates cellular immunity.
Ampligen®	B/D	Altered RNA drug that reduces RNAase levels. Stimulates natural killer cells.
Histamine-2 Blockers	D	These drugs are used mostly as receptor blockers to reduce stomach acid. T Suppressor Cell inhibitors: Tagamet®, Zantac®, Pepcid®, Axid®
Kutapressin	D	A liver extract of peptides which according to anecdotal clinical reports has caused up to a 75% improvement following long-term injection therapy.

ENHANCE ENERGY

Chronic virus infections may cause an adrenal stress which leads to fatigue and hypersensitivity. The nutrients which enhance energy are generally adrenal stimulants which include vitamin C, pantothenic acid, chromium, magnesium, vitamin B-12, vitamin B-6, glandular adrenal, and the herbs: ginseng, gingko biloba, and licorice root.

Medications include Zantac® which enhances energy in many patients, perhaps by blocking the effect of the neurotransmitter histamine on the brain. The use of amphetamines is not recommended due to their addictive tendency, rebound fatigue, and other potentially adverse effects.

ENHANCE COGNITION

Nutrients: B-complex vitamins, phosphatidyl-choline, DMAE, glutamine, and tyrosine. HERBS: Ginseng, gota-cola, schizandra, and ginkgo biloba. The latter increases blood perfusion to the brain, which has been demonstrated in some studies to be low in CFS patients.

Drugs: Hydergine®, Cylert®, piracetam, and other mind-enhancing drugs called "nootropics," many of which are not yet available in the United States but are readily available in Europe. Piracetam and phosphatidylcholine have a potent synergistic quality in enhancing memory and mental capacity in some people.

MOOD DISORDERS

Anti-depressants: Nutrients include phenylalanine, tyrosine and tryptophan. Medications include all the commonly used antidepressants. Prozac®, Elavil®, Wellbutrin®, and Sinequan® are especially helpful. Anti-anxiety nutrients include: calcium and magnesium, vitamin B-6, niacinamide, GABA, taurine and phosphatidyl-choline. Medications: Any appropriate tranquilizer may be used; Klonopin® is especially useful, especially when a marginal seizure disorder is present, due perhaps to the demyelinating brain lesions frequently observed on MRI pictures.

ANTI-INSOMNIA

Nutrients: Tryptophan, calcium, magnesium, selenium, soporific herbs including—chamomile, passion flower, skullcap, valerian, and catnip.

An important note: In recent years tryptophan supplementation has been associated with a condition called Eosinophilia Myalgia syndrome (EMS). Over 1,500 people have developed EMS. However, it has been established that the cause was not the tryptophan itself, but a contaminant that developed in a new process for making this amino acid by a manufacturer in Japan. By 1990, the U.S. government had traced all of the EMS reactions to tryptophan manufactured by a single company in Japan. Recently, Russell M. Jaffe, M.D., Ph.D, has reported on a sucessful series of treatments for patients with EMS in the *International Journal of Biosocial and Medical Research*, which ironically requires uncontaminated (characterized) tryptophan supplements as part of therapy.[3] Currently tryptophan continues to be difficult to procure in most countries, and none is available in the U.S. or Canada over-the-counter, although it has been used successfully in treating depression and sleep disturbances for over 25 million people.

Medications: doxepin has been very helpful in reversing the defect in slow-wave sleep observed in CFS and fibromyalgia. Other hypnotic drugs may be prescribed.

PAIN

Nutrients: All anti-oxidant nutrients may play a role in pain reduction.

Medications: Analgesics as tolerated. Sinequan is especially useful to relieve the pain of fibromyalgia.

Although we have mentioned many general nutrients for these symptoms,we should emphasize the physiologic specificity of nutritional supplementation. It is our theory that the nutrients only work when a person has a deficiency of, or a dependency on, that nutrient. We, therefore, use a lot of trial-and-success (sometimes called trial-and-error). Since nutrients have little pharmacologic (drug-like) action, correction of a health problem with nutrients implies physiologic (natural to the body) action.

BIOLOGICAL RESPONSE MODIFIERS

The current surge of research in immunology has produced exciting developments in the use of nutrients, herbs and biological drugs to modulate the immune response. Immune biologicals are substances manufactured by the human immune system that have been purified and concentrated for medicinal use. Gamma globulin, transfer factor, interleukin-2 and alpha-interferon are examples of biological drugs that offer tremendous promise and hope to people with immune disorders including chronic fatigue syndrome.

GAMMA GLOBULIN

Gamma globulin is a fraction of human blood which contains all the antibodies. Gamma globulin has been available for intramuscular (I.M.) injection for over forty years. This preparation is protective against hepatitis and a wide variety of common infections. It has been used successfully to protect healthcare workers and foreign travelers against hepatitis and other transmissible diseases. In the Persian Gulf war, nearly the entire national stock of I.M. gamma globulin was sent to the Middle East to protect the military against infection.

There are limitations, however, in the uses of I.M. gamma globulin. For one, only small volumes of gamma globulin can be injected into a muscle because the I.M. injections tend to be painful and cause local irritation for several days. One-half to one teaspoon's worth is usually all that can be tolerated at any one time. That amounts to less than a gram of this precious immune fluid in each injection—far too little to help a patient with an immune deficiency.

After many years of research and development a new form of gamma globulin was introduced in the 1980's suitable for intravenous use. Intravenous (I.V.) gamma globulin offers many advantages over the I.M. form. Large quantities of gamma globulin can be administered in a short period of time without local swelling, pain or infection. CFS patients can receive ten to twenty grams of antibodies every week if necessary compared to less than one gram of the I.M. form.

There are two types of disorders that respond to I.V. gamma globulin:

1. Immunodeficiency disorders: either inherited or related to use of immune weakening drugs, malignancies (i.e. leukemias and lymphomas), burns, HIV infection, and CFS. I.V. gamma globulin has been shown to be particularly helpful against the CMV virus.
2. Certain auto-immune diseases, such as idiopathic thrombocytopenic purpura, which is a bleeding disorder, responds very well to IV gamma globulin. Other autoimmune diseases may also respond.

Six American companies manufacture the I.V. preparation. The 3 major companies are: Cutter Laboratories who make *Gammimmune®*, Travenol of the Hyland Corporation, which manufactures *Gammagard®* and Sandoz who produce *Sandoglobin®*. These products are manufactured with strict safety precautions. There is no apparent risk of transmitting hepatitis or HIV retrovirus even though the antibodies are pooled from over ten thousand donors to provide the broadest possible immune protection. These products contain at least 90% of intact gamma globulins with a normal distribution of the IgG subclasses and little or no IgA which could cause serious allergic reactions.

I.V. gamma globulin is generally well tolerated. It is important to infuse this product very slowly, especially during initial use, to prevent side effects like headache, dizziness, nausea and low blood pressure. It is also possible to experience low grade flu symptoms for a day following an infusion.

We believe that the treatment of CFS requires a combined and integrative approach utilizing as many helpful resources as possible. Yet, if we had to select the single most effective treatment for CFS overall, it would have to be gamma globulin. This concentrated pool of antibodies is pre-programmed to intercept and destroy a wide variety of infectious agents including viruses, bacteria and candida. CFS patients tend to have low levels of IgG subclass 1 which, in a healthy person, contains the majority of antibodies against viruses. This antibody fraction is amply supplied by commercial gamma globulin preparations.

The intravenous form of gamma globulin is preferred for use in patients with demonstrable low blood antibody levels, especially if their symptoms are serious and resistant to other types of treatment. However, I.V. gamma globulin is very expensive. The cost of a single infusion is usually between five hundred and one thousand dollars and the average CFS patient requires two to three infusions a month. This is far beyond the means of most people, especially considering that half of all CFS patients are too sick to earn a living. Many subsist on meager and fixed disability income.

Insurance companies have been slow to pick up the tab because they still consider the treatment to be investigational. To have a chance to get insurance coverage, it is important to document every immune defect that is present.

TRANSFER FACTOR

Gamma globulin provides passive immunity. Transfer factor, on the other hand, actively stirs up the immune response. Transfer factor is like an "immune soup." It is a liquid extract of over 100 peptides taken from the lymphocytes of healthy donors. Most of these peptides are presumed to be cytokines capable of influencing immunity. Transfer factor was first described almost fifty years ago when it was noticed that this lymphocyte extract had the ability to transfer a cell-mediated immune response to a microbe from one animal to a recipient animal that had never been exposed to that particular microbe. For example, if the donor had a positive skin test to the measles virus, the recipient would soon develop a positive measles test even though the recipient never had measles. The same immune response could be transferred to a wide variety of viruses, bacteria or yeast organisms.

Transfer factor works on lymphocytes that are early in their maturation, that are still neutral and uncommitted to fighting a specific foe. Under the influence of transfer factor, these lymphocytes rapidly reproduce, mature, and become sensitized.

When transfer factor is injected into people with weak immunity, it can stir up a hornets nest. All facets of the immune response can be involved. Total T cells increase; cytotoxic T cells increase; both T helper and T suppressor cell lines may be stimulated. The effect is broad-based.

It is hard to predict exactly what effect transfer factor will have on a particular patient. The net effect will depend on the specific immune constitutions of both the donor and the recipient. The donor has a unique "immune soup." The recipient has unique immune deficits. What makes transfer factor so special is that it functions like an *adaptogen*. It up regulates immune functions that are suppressed and can down regulate certain autoimmune reactions. Transfer factor should be avoided in patients with connective tissue diseases. It tends to have little effect on a person with a normal, healthy immune response.

Transfer factor has been used clinically to treat stubborn opportunistic viruses in patients with leukemia and other lymphatic cancers. It is also being tried on patients with HIV infection and CFS with some beneficial results, although the salutary effects may take many months to develop. In the early stages of treatment, patients may feel malaise for a day or so following an injection. It is important for patients to commit to a prolonged series of injections of at least six months in duration for optimum benefit.

Unfortunately, transfer factor is not yet available commercially and is not standardized. It is made in private laboratories and in universities. Some insurance companies may still consider it investigational and unsuitable for reimbursement. Most doctors who provide transfer factor initially have patients sign a statement of informed consent.

NUTRITIONAL SUPPLEMENT PROGRAMS

This may turn out to be the most controversial part of this book. To us, as authors, who between us have forty years experience in prescribing nutritional supplement programs in clinical practice, the conventional medical position on nutritional supplementation defies logic. As we have reported in case histories in this book, nutritional supplementation can help to protect us against health hazards inflicted by our polluted environment and dietary practices. Yet, some highly vocal anti-supplement critics stubbornly insist that the American population does not require nutritional supplements. This seems particularly strange given that the U.S. government has committed tens of millions of dollars on reseach on the benefits of various vitamins and minerals in humans. In the U.S. alone there are five major government supported centers at universities conducting voluminous amounts of research on the role of nutrients in human health. Even among dieticians, the majority take nutritional supplements, according to a recently published poll. So it may be reasonable to assume that these highly vocal critics may represent a minority opinion in medicine. The important point is that they continue to shape our perceptions that somehow a doctor choosing to recommend nuritional supplements is suspect.

Our position clearly favors nutritional supplementation as a most powerful weapon in the promotion of health and protection against disease. The medical literature is replete with studies which support our position; there are literally thousands of such research papers. Throughout this chapter and, indeed, in much of this book, we refer to various nutritionally-oriented therapies. In our experience, these modalities are the very cornerstone of treating fatigue from all sources, even in diseases which do not, on the surface, appear to be causally related to nutritional deficiency. The nutritional supplements that boost the immune response are amply described in Chapter Nine: "Nutrition and Immunity".

MISCELLANEOUS INJECTION THERAPIES

The most prominent of these is the intravenous vitamin C drip which may include other injectable vitamins and trace minerals to enhance energy and immunity.

The use of vitamin C infusions originates with the work of the late Fred Klenner M.D. who is one of the unsung heros of medicine. Dr. Klenner, in the small town of Reidsville, North Carolina, discovered the efficacy and safety of IV vitamin C. He practiced and taught his techniques for over forty years and achieved tremendous success in the treatment of refractory infections and auto-immune diseases. His lifeswork was recently published in a fascinating book called the *Clinical Guide to the Use of Vitamin C*. In our experience, intravenous vitamin C is a powerful weapon against CFS. We have seen numerous patients obtain dramatic relief from fatigue and malaise from the use of this modality.

As we have emphasized, the immune system depends on nutrients for its vitality and stability. In this treatment chapter, we specify basic dietary principles and nutritional supplement programs which we use to bolster lagging immunity. Naturally we vary these programs substantially to accommodate the biochemical individuality of our patients.

CONTROVERSIAL INTRAVENOUS THERAPIES

At this time, we should mention other IV therapies which may be pertinent in this condition. Please be clear that these are controversial and have little or no acceptance in conventional medicine. However, there is enough promise and evident safety in these therapies, that they should not be lightly dismissed in dealing with CFS.

1. IV *Chelation Therapy (IVCT)*: Chelation means metal binding. In medicine, chelation therapy (CT) is the primary treatment for metal poisoning. IVCT may improve the immune response by removing toxic heavy metals—such as lead, cadmium, mercury, aluminum, nickel, and arsenic, from the body. It is possible that some CFS patients will require decreasing their body burden of such metals in order to remove the suppression such metals impose on the immune system. EDTA (ethylene diamine tetraacetic acid) is the major chelating agent presently available, but there are many more which may be of great value. There are case reports of patients getting rapid relief from fatigue when undergoing chelation therapy.

2. *Oxidative therapies*: The most curious of the IV therapies has to be hydrogen peroxide (H_2O_2) and its derivatives. Charles Farr, M.D., Ph.D. of Oklahoma City is perhaps the world's leading proponent of this therapy. Dr. Farr researched the literature on oxidative therapies and found that as early as 1924 physicians were successfully using IV H_2O_2 to treat influenza. Dr. Farr found that this therapy both simulates, and stimulates the action of, certain white blood cells in fighting infection. Most physicians do not know that our white blood cells (WBC) produce H_2O_2 as a device to kill invading microorganisms. Simple drugstore hydrogen peroxide, which we use as a topical antiseptic at 3% concentration and a hair bleach at 20%, is also a natural product of the body's immune function. When used as a source of oxidative IV therapy, it is given at 0.03% concentration. Again, the evidence is still anecdotal and far from conclusive, but this therapy may prove to be a viable component of future low toxicity therapy for CFS and other immune dysfunctions. There are dramatic case reports claiming benefits from the use of H_2O_2.

CANDIDA

The idea of candida infection and hypersensitivity causing fatigue incites great controversy in some medical circles. We feel it important to assert that it is a real entity and that Nystatin U.P.S.® oral powder is a key element in treating it. Because of Nystatin's importance, we will digress for a moment to discuss a prominent article in a peer review medical journal, which claims that Nystatin does not work in such cases, and therefore there may be no such disease.

Dr. Dismukes and colleagues published a study in the *New England Journal of Medicine,* which purports to show that Nystatin (a drug that specifically treats certain forms of candida infection) does not work on "possible candida hypersensitivity patients."[1] The study is so flawed that it shocks us to see it published in a leading journal of outstanding reputation. In fact, shortly after its publication, an almost unprecedented number of letters appeared in the same journal criticizing the study. For one thing, the workers in the study did not adequately document the purported candida hypersensitivity in the patients they selected. This in itself is a serious oversight. They did not even test the patients for antibodies to candida, although there are FDA approved clinical tests available. Indeed, they reported no blood studies of any kind. As an additional perplexity, the writers of the article interpreted data opposite to the way they originally reported it at a conference on yeast some two years prior to the publishing of the study. Originally they reported the study as showing positive effects from Nystatin treatment on these patients. Indeed, the data in the published article itself indicates that nystatin worked and, therefore, represents a successful therapeutic trial which supports the notion of a yeast hypersensitivity–fatigue connection. Because of the many flaws in the design and reporting of this study, it becomes necessary to dismiss its negative conclusions. In our experience there is little doubt of the importance of yeast involvement with fatigue. We will therefore proceed to illustrate how we deal with this problem and achieve improvement in a large number of patients.

Treatment of candida yeast infection and hypersensitivity requires a combination of techniques. First and most basic is diet. The anti-yeast diet avoids refined carbohydrates, alcohol and, for many patients, caffeine. Most patients also need to avoid fruit and dairy products (because of the sugar content). The diet consists, therefore, of vegetables, beans, whole grains, poultry, fish and, perhaps, meat. Most doctors who prescribe anti-yeast diets, agree on this part of the diet.

Disagreement occurs among doctors prescribing yeast containing foods such as vinegar and bread. The yeasts in these and other foods bear little resemblance to candida and do not infect humans (as some patients mistakenly believe). Food yeast, however, may cause allergy or hypersensitivity to these yeast containing foods because of cross reaction. Infection with candida increases the likelihood of allergy to the candida and food yeast. The food-yeast, therefore, need not necessarily be excluded from an anti-candida diet unless there is allergy. This allergic cross reaction to candida can trigger allergic rash, with itching and burning, and other allergy phenomena. Food yeast, additionally, contains estrogen like substances which can stimulate candida yeast and make symptoms worse. Some doctors eliminate these yeast-containing foods completely while others only restrict them in patients who are clearly sensitive. Other than these considerations, the diet need not vary much from the basic therapeutic diet presented in this chapter.

The anti-candida diet strategy uses The Basic Therapeutic Diet, with the additional restrictions of fruit, fruit juice, and dairy product.

BASIC THERAPEUTIC DIET

The important aspects of diet concentrate on avoiding empty calorie foods, primarily refined carbohydrates,simple sugars, fatty foods which are high in calories and low in nutrients, and highly processed foods in general. Many patients with yeast infections must also avoid the normally healthful fruits and dairy products.

The Basic Therapeutic Diet is simple in concept and design. It may require some fortitude on the part of those unaccustomed to restricted eating, but most people can learn to follow this kind of eating plan in a month or so. This eating plan even works in restaurants.

The diet approach must account for food allergies and digestive problems. To that end, we also test for food allergies and use an elimination and rotation diet when we suspect food allergies.

This eating plan is designed for simplicity. It makes use of the "wisdom of the body" to manage the amount of food eaten and therefore health and well being. It is best used therapeutically with nutritional supplements.

EMPHASIZE THE FOLLOWING FOODS: (listed by category in order of preference)

1. VEGETABLES AND SPROUTS—artichokes, asparagus, bamboo shoots, beets, broccoli, sprouts, cabbage, carrots, cauliflower, celery, chives, collards, corn, cucumber, eggplant, endive, garlic, Jerusalem artichoke, kale, leeks, lettuce, mushrooms, okra, onions, parsley, parsnips, peas, peppers, pimentos, pumpkin, radish, rutabaga, sauerkraut, spinach, sprouts (alfalfa or bean), squash, sweet potato, swisschard, tomato, turnip, watercress, yams, yeast, zucchini.

2. BEANS AND GRAINS—It is best to combine beans and grains in order to get complete proteins. Always strive for

the least processed and least cooked forms that you can find.

BEANS—Azuki, black, garbonzo (chick-pea), green, lentil, lima, pinto, kidney, yellow wax, white, soy, tofu (soybean protein).

GRAINS AND CEREALS—Barley, corn (including "healthy" popcorn), wheat, rye, brown rice, buckwheat, millet, oatmeal, steelcut oats, tapioca. Bread should be whole wheat or stone ground. Pasta from whole grains or Jerusalem artichoke.

3a. FISH AND SEAFOOD—Abalone, bass, bluefish, carp, catfish, caviar, clam, crab, cod, eel*, flounder, haddock, halibut, herring*, lobster, mackerel*, oyster, perch, pike, pollock, salmon (fresh*), oyster, sardines, scallops, shad*, shrimp, smelt, snails, snapper, swordfish**, trout*, tuna**, wakeme, whitefish*.

3b. POULTRY—Chicken, duck*, goose*, pheasant, turkey, chicken liver and liver pate. hen's eggs*.

(*high fat, **high mercury)

4. FRUITS—Fresh preferable; frozen is acceptable, avoid canned or dried as much as possible.
Apple, apricot, avocado, berries, cherries, citrus (especially grapefruit), melons, nectarine, pear, peach, pineapple, papaya, mango, tangerine.

Avoid bananas, plums, grapes, prunes, and other dried fruit

5. NUTS AND SEEDS—Good for snacks and good protein source. (Note: Relatively high in fats.)

6. DAIRY—Many people do better with none at all. Yogurt, buttermilk, and other acidophilus digested products are best.

7. (RED) MEAT—Limit to two servings per week because of fat and additives. Avoid processed meats such as sausage, ham, and bacon. Lamb, liver, veal, beef, venison, rabbit, pork.

BEVERAGES—Herb tea and pure non-tap water are the best. Freshly juiced carrots, celery and other vegetables are excellent. Seltzer and club soda are okay. Fruit juices are best avoided for people with poor energy or possible yeast infections; many people get sugar reactions from fruit juice.

DESSERTS—Unsweetened gelatin, fruit, whole grain (honey-sweetened) pastry.

TOTALLY AVOID—Alcohol beverages. Caffeine: tea & coffee (including decaf), chocolate, cola, etc.. All refined sugars (including glucose, fructose, fruit sugar, dextrose, dextrins, corn sweeteners, Barbados molasses, blackstap molasses, buttered syrup, caramel, carob syrup, dextran, dextrose, diastase, diastatic malt, ethyl maltol, honey, maple syrup, molasses, saccharin, sorbitol, sucrose, turbinado sugar, etc.). Foods containing added sugars. Especially avoid candy, pastry, pudding, ice cream.

Potato (acts like fruit).

Refined Carbohydrates: breads and pastas made with white flour (enriched, bleached, etc.), white rice. Chewing gum (even "sugar-free"). Watch out, Nutrasweet® (aspartame) artificial sweetener has been reported by the U.S. Center for Disease Control to cause a wide range of neurological reactions, including depression and fatigue, in previously symptom-free people. Simple cessation of this artificial sweetener eliminates symptoms in 7-10 days.

GENERAL CONSIDERATIONS

1. Butter, preferably unsalted, is better than margarine.
2. Learn not to add excess salt. The civilized diet is generally loaded with it. But people with low stomach acid sometimes need to have moderate salt.
3. Salad dressings should be clear oil not creamy, apple cider vinegar (if you have no vinegar sensitivity), and lemon or lime. Spices and herbs are good.
4. Snacks: carrots, celery, radish, mushrooms, seeds, nuts, salad veges.
5. Liver may be the most nourishing all-around food, even though it may contain toxins—everything contains toxins, but not everything has redeeming virtues.
6. Sprouts are probably the most wholesome foods.

7. Cabbage, kale, and brussel sprouts may be a little hard on the digestive system and the thyroid gland. They bind iodine. Generally do not eat more than twice weekly.
8. All artificial sweeteners, particularly aspartame (Nutra-Sweet®) are probably best avoided. They are chemical flavor enhancers of no nutritive value.
9. Soups should be clear, not creamy. Beware of high salt, sugar, and grain fillers.
10 "Wheat bread" is a deceptive term; it means processed wheat flour which has been colored brown. Always be sure the label says *whole wheat* or *stone ground.*
11. *YEAST is only dangerous to those who are allergic to it.* Otherwise it is nourishing. Most people do well with it. *This includes those who have Candida infections,* as long as they are not allergic to that specific yeast.
12. In general, eat as close to nature as possible—raw whenever that is palatable. Tend to undercook. Vegetables crisp rather than soggy. Avoid using a pressure cooker.
13. Eggs have high cholesterol but also high nourishment. They should be eaten soft-boiled, poached, or hard-boiled. Scrambled eggs and omelettes expose the cholesterol to heat, oxygen, and metal which damages the cholesterol by oxidizing it.

The diet approach must consider food allergy and digestive disturbances resulting from dysfunction of the organs which provide for the digestive enzymes and other agents essential to the digestive process. To that end, we will address the provocative food testing program with the use of the rotation diet when we suspect food allergy.

The patient, as already stated, should avoid any food which may be causing allergy or sensitivity; this often includes yeast and vinegar. The allergy problem in candida may ambush the unsuspecting victim.

In supplementing the candida CFS patient, we start with the basic supplement plan and individualize according to the patient's need. The basic plan is simple and sometimes delightfully dramatic. The sudden improvement in many of these sufferers amazes us constantly. The simplicity of the process defies our medical school education which says that such response is placebo or some misplaced enthusiasm. When we increase the sophistication of the nutritional program with our decades of nutritional experience, we see increased power in the supplementation.

We recommend the use of anti-oxidants in candida infections.

NUTRIENT YEAST KILLERS

A number of natural yeast killers have surfaced since the revelations about yeast in recent years. Caprylic acid and other medium chain fatty acids have led the way in much of this battle. These fatty acids which derive from such sources as coconuts, olives, and castor beans, have demonstrated clinical effectiveness against candida. They achieve greatest effect when given in conjunction with a complete program. Many patients report excellent control of symptoms on these preparations.

Garlic, the folk remedy which harks back to Hippocrates, reveals its effectiveness in many ways. It contains allicin as well as other sulfur compounds which seem to suppress yeast and other invaders. With few side effects, garlic can suppress and contain many infections. Pure Gar® and Kwai® are brands of deodorized garlic available through over 100 supplement manufactures world-wide.

Acidophilus (*Lactobacillus acidophilus*) often anchors the defense against yeast. It certainly occupies an important role in the flora of the human bowel.[2] Acidophilus is the primary natural supplement for recolonizing a dysbiotic (or imbalanced) bowel flora. Imbalance of the normal bowel flora results from overuse of antibiotics, steroid hormones, and overconsumption of such food-stuffs as sugar and alcohol. This dysbiosis can be alleviated by reintroducing these organisms into the bowel. A confusing aspect of this therapy is the many inadequate lactobacillus preparations on the market. Often patients need to change brands, doses and formulations of acidophilus in order to get the desirable effect. We have laboratory tested several brands for potency, and found some that are very effective and reliable, the NCFM strain being a particularly good probiotic. The effect becomes obvious when the patient demonstrates a dramatic improvement of symptoms. Gas, cramps, diarrhea, or constipation may disappear almost overnight. Fatigue itself may diminish due to use of a viable L. *acidophilus* supplement.

We sometimes add other forms of lactobacillus, such as L. *bulgaricus*, because they may improve the therapeutic effect that acidophilus gives us, but we do not give them in the same preparation. Using combinations may work at cross purposes because the different species may interfere with one another, each giving off componds to control the growth of its competition. We, therefore, use individual preparations of the different bacilli at different times. Avoid using combination products.

Numerous other modalities contribute to suppressing overgrowth of candida. Herbs such as golden seal, shiitake mushrooms, mathaki, pau d'arco tea, and others may all be beneficial. Paracan, the oil from the grapefruit seed, has a powerful herb-like action on candida, as does tannic acid which is available in commercial preparations. Tannic acid, by the way, is the substance that supposedly makes the Okefenokee Swamp (Florida) water a popular therapeutic folk remedy to the locals who live there. A large array of biological therapies can attack candida. We do not use nearly all that are available or potentially beneficial. For example, consider the vast number of Chinese herbs which many practitioners of Oriental medicine use, and with which we are only beginning to become familiar in North America and Europe.

ANTI-FUNGAL DRUGS

We use antifungal drugs with mixed emotions. We would wish to avoid such drugs whenever possible. Yet, we find that often these drugs can produce fast and safe cures of yeast infection. The three main drugs which we employ in this situation are Nystatin®, ketoconazole (Nizoral®), and fluconazole (Diflucan®).

Nystatin: Oral nystatin powder can effectively suppress candida overgrowth in the bowel. We also use it topically on skin and vaginal yeast infections. It has virtually no toxicity when used topically, orally, or vaginally. It may cause die-off reactions or allergy which give side effects that are unpleasant but not dangerous. It can have distinct effects on systemic candidiasis when used orally. We have found, incidentally, that other forms of Nystatin such as tablets or alcohol based solutions have much less effectiveness in candidiasis. This fact has actually served as a sort of control in our experience. We have seen patients who for one reason or another have used the Nystatin tablets, fully believing that form of nystatin would be therapeutic. In many cases, there was no therapeutic response until they switched to the Nystatin powder. The powder is harder to find in most pharmacies, less convenient to use, and somewhat more expensive. We like the powder only because it works much better.

Ketoconazole (Nizoral®): When Nystatin fails or does not seem appropriate for other reasons, we will advance to Nizoral (or Diflucan®). Nizoral absorbs through the intestinal wall when taken orally, and traverses the blood stream, thereby penetrating anywhere there may be invasive yeast. Nizoral would seem preferable to Nystatin if it did not carry the risk of liver toxicity. It can attack the liver to different degrees, depending on the individual's susceptibility. The side effect commonly noticed with Nizoral is nausea. This may progress to severe malaise, with intestinal pain. In severe cases, jaundice appears as a chemical hepatitis develops and the liver dysfunctions. Dangerous reactions can occur. However rare, these reactions cause us to use Nizoral sparingly and with great vigilance. We take blood samples frequently, especially during the first few months, in order to monitor the condition of the liver. The power of Nizoral to cure nystatin-resistant patients keeps it in our armamentarium despite the difficulty in using it.

Fluconazole (Diflucan®): Diflucan became available in early 1990. It would seem that the only reason to use Nizoral now that Diflucan exists is economics. Diflucan costs several times more than Nizoral. At about $15.00 per pill for the 200 mg. dose, a one month treatment costs in the neighborhood of $450.00. Some people get by with half that amount. When the patient can afford Diflucan, the results often delight us. It surpasses by far the effectiveness of Nystatin and Nizoral. It does so with a minimum of toxicity. Again, we have seen many patients with candidiasis fail to respond to or tolerate Nystatin or Nizoral, but respond quickly to Diflucan. We should note that we had a number of such patients in the Spring of 1990 when Diflucan first became available. In many of these patients, Diflucan was the calvary arriving to save the day. Despite its cost, we are grateful it is on the market.

CANDIDA HYPERSENSITIVITY AND DESENSITIZATION

Allergy desensitization therapy, such as shots used for hay fever, are sometimes useful in the treatment of candida hypersensitivity. Many candida patients develop a true allergy to the yeast. This response can manifest as fatigue with itching and burning of the skin and vaginal discharge. This discharge may not contain yeast on laboratory testing. In recent years, researchers discovered, in the vaginal discharge, IgE antibodies (which cause allergies to candida). Candida infection and allergy, therefore, may coexist or may occur separately. Treating the infection may reduce the hypersensitivity response but may not clear it completely. This explains why some women with candida-like vaginitis may have no sign of infection. They may not respond to treatment with vaginal suppositories because there is no yeast infection. It is an allergy. Accordingly, we often have the patient undergo allergy skin testing to determine the antigen dose to relieve candida hypersensitivity. This test is simple and straightforword.

We observe that yeast often coexists with food allergies. We, therefore, need to include diet in the treatment plan because of the cross allergic phenomenon. This means that the development of an allergy to candida yeast can lead to a cross reaction with yeast in food.

Fortunately, this does not occur most of the time, but the possibility requires vigilance. We sometimes utilize several aspects of dietary management—namely, avoidance, challenge, and rotation types of diets. This means that we have patients avoid suspected allergic foods for at least four days, then add back the suspected foods one at a time and see if the foods provoke symptoms with the challenge. That approach identifies the culprits and leads to the rotation diet. The rotation diet minimizes the likelihood of developing more allergies. Allergies beget more allergies. As allergy increases demands on the immune system, the system's ability to function normally becomes more impaired. It can reach a point where the allergies become an avalanche. The patient then may become a "universal reactor" or "environmental illness" (EI) victim. And victim is the right word. Few disease states so overwhelm a patient. The patient becomes a prisoner of the world. Common inhalants, most foods, fabrics, sometimes even sunlight or cold temperatures can trigger debilitating reactions. These patients constantly react to their daily environment. We mention this here because candidiasis and CFS may ultimately lead to EI in some people.

PARASITES

Most doctors treat parasites with drugs. We feel that treating parasitic infection begins with the immune system. We, therefore, refer you to the diagnostic flow sheet and the diet and immune boosting supplements in the appendix. With those in place, we consider specific treatments for parasites. We use, for this purpose, both medical drugs and natural herbs. We use them separately or together, depending on the circumstance. The patient's preference and apparent ability to tolerate medications determine the choices. If, on the one hand, the patient abhors drugs of any kind and has no great urgency to be rid of a chronic pest with low grade symptomatology, we opt for herbal treatment. If, on the other hand, the patient feels fine with the idea of drug therapy, wants a quick and more certain result, and has concern about the non-scientific nature of herbal treatment, medication clearly wins the decision. Much of the time we find situations in between these extremes; we then may employ combinations of drugs and herbs.

STOOL SPECIMENS (PURGE TEST)
READ INSTRUCTIONS CAREFULLY BEFORE STARTING

These are the instructions which we have developed for our stool purge patients. They have been edited many times to answer questions that arise during the procedure and are self explanatory.

The purpose of the stool purge is to get the best possible sample of bowel parasites and yeast. The routine random stool tests being done in standard labs are generally not adequate for our needs and do not get medically useful results.

Dietary instructions:

1. Light meal the evening prior to the purge; drink only clear liquids (water, herb tea, etc.)
2. No breakfast the morning of the purge.
3. Best results are from morning purges, but that is not essential.
4. Bring specimen to office within two days or mail it (C/O Office Lab) as soon as possible. **(Note: There is a preservative in the specimen bottle. Be careful not to spill it. There is no need to refrigerate the specimen.)**

The objective of the stool purge is to secure a watery, "explosive" sample. This gives far better reliability than numerous random samples. It pulls organisms out of the tissues so that they may be diagnosed. **If the specimen is thicker than watery, its reliability decreases.** It usually takes three to six bowel movements to produce the watery sample. The following procedure will usually achieve that result. Some people may have to vary the procedure, but the instructions will cover most situations.

Note: Do not do purge within 24 hours prior to blood testing; it will distort the blood test.

1. Drink entire 1 1/2 ounces of Fleet's Phospho-Soda laxative (provided.) Children, seriously ill people, or people with diarrheal conditions should take proportionately less. In such case, consult your doctor for individual instruction.
2. Discard first five bowel movements. Typically, this will take about two hours. Some labs ask for the third bowel movement.
3. If explosive, obviously watery bowel movement occurs earlier, it is okay to use that specimen.

4. Place a collection bowl in the toilet so that you can catch the sixth bowel movement. If it is not watery, take only 1/2 specimen and wait for later BM's to become watery. If the process is dragging on past two hours, you may take 1/2 specimen from a less watery sample, then wait for the watery sample which may occur later. Then fill the rest of the specimen bottle.
5. Use the disposable dropper to stir the specimen lightly and draw up a mixed portion of the specimen.
6. Fill the specimen bottle within 1/2 inch of the top. Secure lid firmly. **The preservative is formalin and is mildly irritating to skin and very much so to eyes. If any splashes on you, flush copiously with water.**
7. Put your name and your doctor's name on the label and return it to our office as directed above.

Please allow seven working days for the results. If your have an appointment to discuss the test, please confirm that the test results are ready before you come in.

Remember, no purge for 24 hours prior to blood work.

ANTI-PARASITIC DRUGS

Although there are many more drugs than we mention here, the drugs in the section give us the best service. They provide the best ratio of therapeutics to toxicity. This section could be much expanded, especially when we look around the world at drugs not available because of USA regulation.

Metronidazole (Flagyl): This drug which kills ameba (*Entameba histolytica*) and trichomonas (*Trichomonas vaginalis*) is also useful in treating Giardia (*Giardia lamblia*). It has a broad spectrum of activity against protozoal parasites as well as powerful antibiotic qualities against certain important anaerobic bacterial pathogens. In standard doses it has intestinal side effects such as nausea, cramping, malaise, and sometimes vomiting; when used according to standard guidelines, it is fairly safe. It could be considered the preeminent drug in protozoal and anaerobic bacterial therapeutics.

We use metronidazole for Giardia in standard doses. We also use it for E. *histolytica* (Amebiasis), but in combination with Yodoxin® (diiodoquinol). Ameba therapy usually requires both these drugs because of the nature of the intestinal infection and the pharmacology of the two drugs. Ameba (E. *histolytica*) lives in the wall of the intestine as well as the lumen. In order to treat this situation effectively, we must give drugs which concentrate in both areas. Unfortunately, no single drug presently fills that requirement. Metronidazole totally concentrates in the blood stream and tissues, being completely absorbed in the small intestine. Conversely, Yodoxin remains totally in the lumen of the bowel, since it is virtually unabsorbed. When used in concert, the drugs have a high success rate eradicating E. *histolytica* from the patient.

We also use metronidazole to treat G. *lamblia*. This common protozoa which is endemic in practically the entire world, responds well to standard dose metronidazole without concomitant use of Yodoxin.

Metronidazole has activity against *Trichomonas vaginalis* which may not play a major role in the fatigue picture. Nevertheless, when we treat T. *vaginalis* or any of the other wide range of organisms which metronidazole attacks, we get a two edged sword or—in this case, perhaps a sword that cuts three ways. First, we have the benefit of killing many pathogenic organisms. Second, we have the problem of killing many friendly microorganisms, thereby allowing for possible yeast or parasite opportunistic overgrowth. Third, we have the toxicity of the drug which may be from the drug itself or may be from the Herxheimer reaction, sometimes called "die-off." Herxheimer, releases toxins from the dying organisms which can suddenly increase the symptoms which usually come from the steady state of the organism with a lower rate of toxin release. Thus, two of the reactions create harm, with the added difficulty of distinguishing between them. Notwithstanding the reactions, the effectiveness of the treatment more than mitigates the side effects in most cases. We have participated in many successful cases with iodoquinol combined with metronidazole.

Iodoquinol (Yodoxin®): This drug occupies a rather obscure niche in U.S. pharmacology. It may not be on every pharmacist's shelf, but it is available with a little persistence. Usually, the pharmacist must special order it. We stock it in our office for patient convenience. We use it for the reasons already mentioned regarding adequate treatment of E. *histolytica*. Yodoxin also carries the added benefit of relatively low toxicity and side effect when used for short courses of treatment. We generally use it for twenty days. We find that patients tolerate it well.

Quinacrine hydrochloride (Atabrine®): Quinicrine is a venerable parasite killer, the use of which goes back to World War II. While it cures giardial infections, its major use has been with malaria which probably does not pertain to CFS—at least in the United States. When used in a CFS patient with proven giardia, it works well although it can cause liver toxicity and can turn the skin yellow in susceptible individuals. The yellow skin from Atabrine is not from jaundice. It has its own vivid pigment which makes it undesirable in those who respond with yellow skin. It has also been used with some success in the treatment of amebiasis.

Mebendazole (Vermox®): Mebendazole eliminates common roundworms (*Ascaris lumbricoides*) and pinworms (*Enterobius vermicularis*) as well as other helminths. We find common roundworms responding well to this treatment. We use the recommended dose and repeat it in seven days, thus increasing the chance of resolving the infection.

Furazolidone (Furoxone®): Furoxone gives us a good alternative in the treatment of giardia and some intestinal bacterial infections. Patients tolerate it well. The side effects are definite but well understood, predictable, and usually mild.

Paramomycin (Humatin®): We have not used this drug much, but mention it as an alternative to Yodoxin in the treatment of amebiasis. Humatin is indicated for intestinal amebiasis, especially in the carrier state, but like Yodoxin, it will not penetrate the tissues. Humatin, therefore will not treat invasive amebiasis. It seems usefulness as an adjunct to metronidazole or for the individual who is in the carrier state.

This somewhat incomplete array of medications applies mostly to our experience in the USA; other antiparasitics certainly apply to rare occurrences. We saw one patient in whom we managed to discover dwarf tapeworm (Hymenolepsis nana). This nasty parasite, usually found in tropical climates, can cause serious consequences. We treated it successfully with Niclocide® (niclosamide.) We have only had two occasions to use that drug. It may be widely useful in some parts of the world, but obviously we only mention it as an example of a treatment with small statistical value to us. Many other medications exist around the world, just as many diseases which are uncommon to us. We wish that we had access to some of the other medications, but our U.S. Food and Drug Agency (FDA) does not allow them.

A fairly large number of our patients have foregone the drug route for the herbal-nutritional approach. Our general experience is that many of them succeed and many do not. It is hard to put a statistic on it, but it is probably about 50-50. Those who succeed without drugs avoid the side effects which bother a majority who take the medications. The non-drug, purely nutritional approach usually takes considerably longer and does not give the high likelihood of quick success which we get with medications. Most of our patients opt for the combination nutrient-drug routine, suffer the physical upsets which are manageable, and get well much quicker.

The most widely used herb among the many hundreds available, is probably artemesia annua (wormwood). This venerable preparation seems to suppress protozoa such as ameba and giardia. It also seems to have effectiveness against Cryptosporidium, the parasite which probably contributes to the CFS of some patients, but has not yet gained official acceptance as being the cause of any chronic disease state. Artemesia seems to have eliminated Cryptosporidium in some of our patients. These patients have, however, also taken our immune diet and supplement program.

TREATMENT SCHEDULE FOR ANTI-PARASITIC DRUGS

The parasite treatment plan is designed to reduce the likelihood of developing a "die-off" reaction to the powerful antiparasitic treatment we are prescribing. By starting at a low dose, and gradually increasing, as tolerated by the patient, the risk of serious reaction can be almost eliminated.

The two drugs used are Yodoxin (iodoquinol) and metronidazole (Flagyl). There are many treatment schedules possible with these agents. There are also many adjunctive therapies that can be used. Here is a general plan that will fit the majority of our patients. For many of you, we may modify this outline to suit your individual needs.

WARNING: These drugs can cause serious side effects including skin reactions, intestinal upset, headaches, thyroid reactions, and liver toxicity. Allergic reactions of any kind are possible. If you develop any unexplained reaction during use of these drugs, stop using them and phone your physician for advice.

Metronidazole should never be used with any alcohol consumption.

Iodoquinol (Yodoxin®) 650mg. **Metronidazole** (Flagyl®) 250mg.

DAY		AM	MID	PM		AM	MID	PM
1		1	1	1		0	0	0
2	<-->	1	1	1	<------>	0	0	0
3		1	1	1		1	0	0
4	<-->	1	1	1	<------>	1	0	1
5		1	1	1		1	1	1
6	<-->	1	1	1	<------>	2	1	1
7		1	1	1		2	1	2
8	<-->	1	1	1	<------>	2	2	2
9		1	1	1		2	2	2
10	<-->	1	1	1	<------>	2	2	2
11		1	1	1		2	2	2
12	<-->	1	1	1	<------>	2	2	2
13		1	1	1		2	2	2
14	<-->	1	1	1	<------>	0	0	0
15								
16								
17								
18		DAYS 15 THROUGH 20, REPEAT DAY 14						
19								
20								

(Dosage based on 70 kilogram person. Adjust up or down according to weight.)

This plan gives a total of 20 days of Yodoxin at 3 per day which totals 60 caps.

It gives a total of 51 of the 250 mg metronidazole.

The reason for using this approach in the treatment of amebiasis, is that no single drug will reliably and simultaneously destroy the two populations of ameba which infect the bowel wall as well as the hollow in the bowel (called the lumen.) Yodoxin is effective in the lumen, while metronidazole is effective in the bowel wall itself. Together they can accomplish total destruction of the ameba, which neither can do alone.

BACTERIA

Treating the bacteria involved in the CFS/CF problem may range from simple to extremely difficult. If we seek and find an occult bacterial infection in a patient labeled with CFS, we treat that person with the appropriate antibiotic, standard medicine prevails, and there is little need for us to dwell on it here. In the ideal case, treated conventionally, the physician finds and cultures a sample of the bacteria causing the infection. The culture and bacterial sensitivity studies then give the physician a selection of antibiotic choices with which to treat. Given that scenario, the process often succeeds in ridding the patient of the infection. If the infection has caused the fatigue, the patient will be well.

Several perplexities may complicate this idyllic scene:

1. An infection may not be found. This misfortune may result from a physician's not being aggressive enough in his diagnostic work-up. Another explanation may be the patient's unwillingness to do what the physician asks. This problem obviously stems from diagnostics rather than treatment, but the treatment of bacterial infections has more direct relationship with the diagnosis than most medical conditions.

   Finding the exact bacterial organism and its location rates among the most satisfying things we can do as physicians. The physician's responsibility here includes aggressively seeking the diagnosis and communicating effectively with the patient to achieve cooperation and a team approach. That accomplished, many hidden infections often emerge. We find infections of the prostate, tonsils, kidneys, teeth, sinuses, lungs—to name a few of the most commonly found. Such infections may lurk beneath the surface and require more diagnostic effort than ordinary medicine has available. There may be other even more perplexing bacterial infections such as Lyme disease, a tick-borne spirochetal infection, which may defy ordinary diagnostics.

2. Once found, extraordinary infections may require extraordinary therapy. Hippocrates said: *Drastic conditions require drastic remedies.* Sometimes patients with such infections may need to have two or three times the ordinary dose of antibiotics for five or ten times the ordinary course. It takes a lot of thought to venture out and design individualized programs in such cases. Instead of a 7 day treatment for vaginitis every few weeks, it may require an unorthodox 28 consecutive days. Over twenty years ago Thomas McPherson Brown, M.D., at George Washington University, treated his rheumatoid arthritis (RA) patients with antibiotics for 10 or 11 months! He reported 60% improvement in a disease which today most doctors still

do not recognize as possibly being infectious. That makes Dr. Brown an unacknowledged visionary if he was right or wildly irresponsible enthusiast if he was wrong. RA patients are obviously not CFS victims, but they uniformly have fatigue and malaise, and the late Dr. Brown was unique in his approach. If he truly got people better by venturing forth from the fold, we need to consider that type of approach in certain individuals. This discussion points up the need to be creative and imaginative with bacterial infections which may be involved with CFS.

3. We cannot ignore the problems caused by the antibiotics. What are the complications of giving even ordinary amounts of antibiotics, not to mention the extraordinary approaches we just mentioned? Certainly there can be enormous repercussions from the use of antibiotics. Antibiotics can cause allergic reactions some of which can be lethal; some antibiotics have direct toxicity to liver, kidney, nervous system, etc. Perhaps most important, antibiotics lead to overgrowth of yeast and normally innocuous bacteria in the body. Antibiotics may actually be the major cause of chronic candida infection which in turn may lead to CFS. Remember what we said about antibiotic treatment of acne leading to yeast infestation and subsequent candida hypersensitivity syndrome. We need to remember the use of the friendly bacteria from the Lactobacillus family to minimize the risk of yeast and secondary bacterial overgrowth. As mentioned before, acidophilus may provide the best single protection against bacterial and yeast overgrowth associated with antibiotic therapy. Vitamin A, and vitamin C, zinc, and selenium, are some of the nutrients which boost the immune system.

STRESS MASTERY
(Through Consciousness)

This information, plus some of the discussion in Chapter 7, parallels the Stress Mastery tape which we often recommend to our patients. The tape provides the background which will give information and understanding about stress. It also provides a guided exercise with which a person can learn to confront, bring to consciousness, and hence master the stress response. The discussion here does not go into the same exact approach, but may give enough information to allow a diligent reader to increase his or her mastery of stress.

To begin with:

Four basic emotions create the stress response which is triggered by the mind. All emotions fit into one of these categories which are: Glad—Mad—Sad—Scared.

In outline form, here some of the synonyms for those four emotions.

A. Glad (love)—happiness, joy, lightheartedness, exhilaration, elation, euphoria, exaltation, ecstasy, enthusiasm, gaiety, brightness, cheer, radiance, affection, endearment.

B. Mad (anger)—rage, frustration, ire, indignation, wrath, umbrage, pique, provocation, irritation, aggravation, gall, exasperation, riled.

C. Sad (depression)—melancholy, mournfulness, lugubrious, somber, unhappiness, gloom, sorrow, rue, woe, bleakness, desolation, lamentation, dolefulness.

D. Scared (fear)—tension, anxiety, terror, nervousness, jittering, jumpiness, spookiness, fright, concern, worry, consternation, alarm, dread, uneasiness, uptight, edginess, panic, petrified.

Subjectively, we experience much of this response in our muscles. For all the words that we have to describe these relatively simple muscular sensations, they fit into three categories

I. Sensations (simple — musculo-skeletal system):
   Pressure
   Temperature
   Movement

There are more complex sensations which create stressful demands on us, but these complex emotions do not interfere with this simple approach to the stress of CFS. We still work with the three simple musculo-skeletal sensations. For the record, here are some of the sensations with which we do not work directly. When we work with the three basic sensations of muscular stress, we find that the excess stress response to the more complex sensations gets softened.

Sensations (complex):

Hunger	Nausea
Sex	Itch
Pleasure	Tickled
Pain	

Besides Selye, the most influential workers in our concept of stress were Pavlov and Freud. Pavlov discovered the conditioned reflex by stimulating dogs with food and bells. With food, the dogs salivated; with bells they did not. However, after stimulating the dogs with food and bells simultaneously enough times, the dogs became conditioned to the bells and would salivate with just them and without the food. He then could expand that response to bells and buzzers and develop a second order response without the food. In the laboratory, Pavlov could not get beyond a third order response. It may be that human behavior is so complex that it could develop multi-order responses. Even if humans can only develop third order responses, this could lead to stress response from stimuli that seemingly have nothing to do with the original cause of the stress. If a child gets frightened by his parents at the dinner table enough times, it could lead to second order stress response to food or kitchen tables or a certain color of wall paint. There is little question that we have free floating stress response to such mysterious, repressed stimuli.

Repression is the other key concept. It may well be that Freud's most important contribution to science is the theory that repressed memories in the unconscious cause psychological problems. Much of Freud's work and the subsequent psychology and psychiatry techniques which have evolved since Freud work at unrepressing these subconscious, painful memories. Once such a memory is brought to consciousness, its power to disturb the individual diminishes or disappears. Freud and others accomplish this task by analyzing and confronting these memories.

We employ a similar technique in our approach to stress management. We recommend a technique which enlightens the patient about the stress response, both didactically and experientially. We use a stress tape which explains and defines stress in simple terms on the first side. On the second side is a 12 minute exercise which allows the patient to explore the sensations in the muscles when in a stressful circumstance. After practicing this exercise enough times, most people get proficient enough to do the technique in a few seconds—anywhere, anytime. This technique can effectively unrepress the present. It seems that conditioned reflexes, like repressed memories, can be deconditioned by consciousness of the process. If we can increase the patient's consciousness, the patient may then master the stress response.

II. Method

A. Scan the body as soon as the stressful demand hits you.

B. Focus quickly and clearly on every sensation that results from the stress response.

C. Notice that the stressful response fades with increased consciousness of the body sensations.

III. Ergo: Stress Mastery——Unrepressing the Present.

A. Practice reviewing your bodily sensations.

B. Become adept at quickly scanning your entire body for the physical response to stress—even though your mind wants to block it out. The more conscious you are of your body sensations, the more mastery. The realization of each body response allows it to disappear. Being able to do this simple technique gives you the power to overcome the conditioned response. The conditioned response is totally unconscious.

It should be possible to achieve this mastery to the degree that one can reduce stress in a few seconds by quickly scanning the body response and having the consciousness of the stress response allow the stress consequences to disappear.

Consciousness is the path to mastery.

COMPLETION

We have been blessed with wide success in treating our patients, many of whom were beleaguered by their frustrating diseases. How we treat the failures may ultimately provide the key to the enigma. We continue our quest in concert with the scientific community, seeking this elusive phantom. It is our mission to continue to work with the scientific community and our patients until there emerges a final solution to the frustration of the chronic fatigue syndrome.

We believe that research will soon locate most of the missing pieces to the puzzle of Chronic Fatigue Syndrome. Our quest for these solutions continues, but no one, as of this date, can claim an ultimate solution. In addition to the solutions we have discussed, we always consider many more possibilities. Homeopathy and acupuncture certainly get results in many patients. Additionally, much of the nutritional treatment which we have done is akin to Naturopathy, but Naturopathy can further offer some of its own unique possibilities—just as can Chiropractic and some forms of body work. Psychology, psychiatry, and other forms of behavioral therapy can be vital to many CFS patients. Our focus on nutritional, medicinal, and injectable therapies has purposely ignored may of these other valuable modalities. We certainly work in close concert with many practitioners from all of these disciplines. We chose not to explore and explain these approaches for now, since our approach already touched on so many diverse areas. It is now clear to us that there needs to be an even more comprehensive book which includes details of how these various disciplines can interact successfully.

We wish you health and energy.

REFERENCES

1. Dismukes, W.E., *et al.* A randomized, double-blind trial of nystatin therapy for the candidiasis hypersensitivity syndrome. *New Eng J Med.*, 1990; 323.
2. Schauss, A.G. Lactobacillus acidophilus: Method of action, clinical application, and toxicity data. *J Advance Med.*, 1990; 3: 163-178.
3. Jaffe, R.E. Eosinophilia-myalgia syndrome caused by contaminated tryptophan. *Int J Bios Med Res.*, 1990; 11: 181-184.

APPENDIX

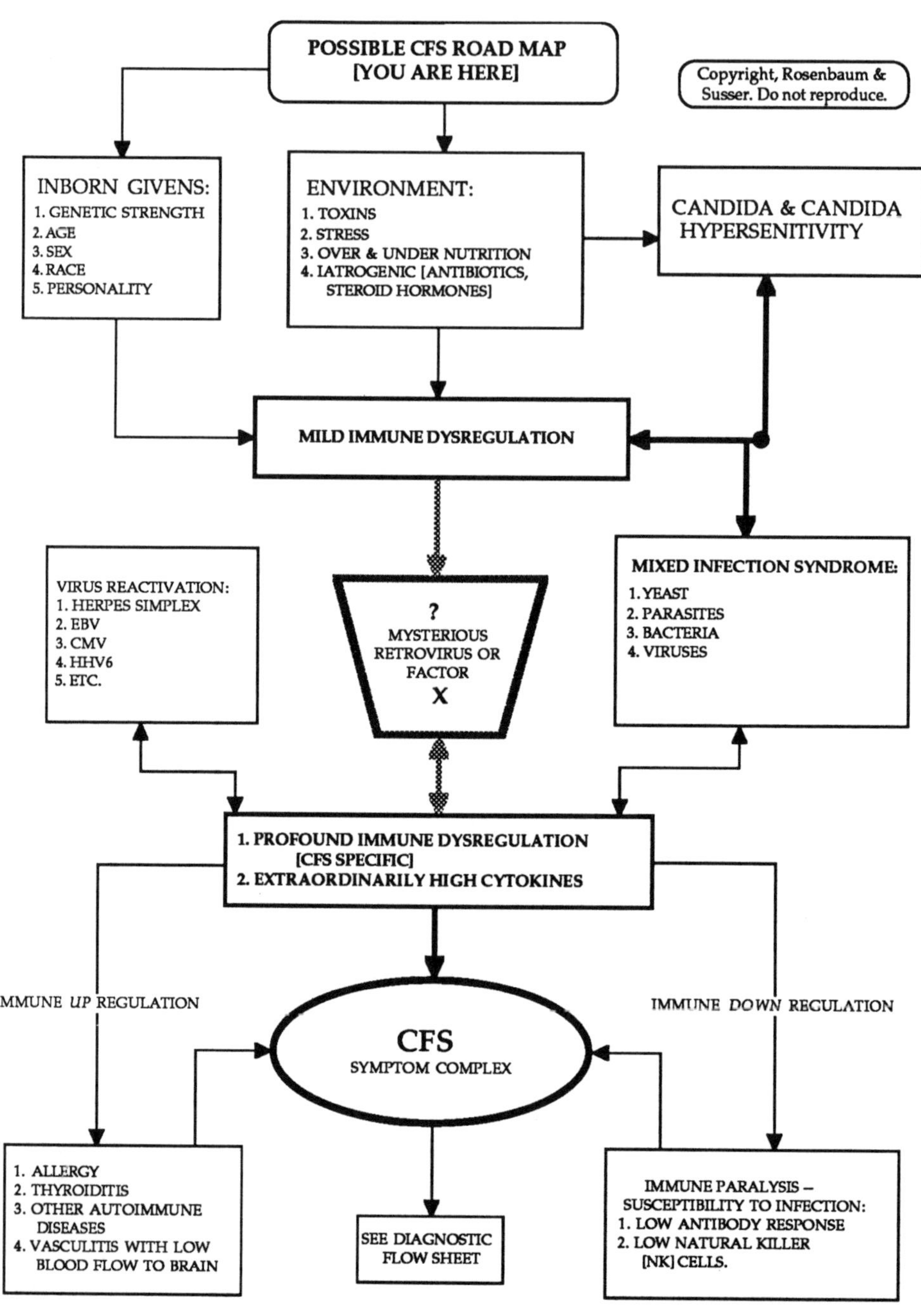

POSSIBLE CFS ROAD MAP
[YOU ARE HERE]
Copyright, Rosenbaum & Susser. Do not reproduce.
INBORN GIVENS:
1. GENETIC STRENGTH
2. AGE
3. SEX
4. RACE
5. PERSONALITY
ENVIRONMENT:
1. TOXINS
2. STRESS
3. OVER & UNDER NUTRITION
4. IATROGENIC [ANTIBIOTICS, STEROID HORMONES]
CANDIDA & CANDIDA HYPERSENITIVITY
MILD IMMUNE DYSREGULATION
VIRUS REACTIVATION:
1. HERPES SIMPLEX
2. EBV
3. CMV
4. HHV6
5. ETC.
?
MYSTERIOUS RETROVIRUS OR FACTOR
X
MIXED INFECTION SYNDROME:
1. YEAST
2. PARASITES
3. BACTERIA
4. VIRUSES
1. PROFOUND IMMUNE DYSREGULATION [CFS SPECIFIC]
2. EXTRAORDINARILY HIGH CYTOKINES
IMMUNE UP REGULATION
IMMUNE DOWN REGULATION
CFS
SYMPTOM COMPLEX
1. ALLERGY
2. THYROIDITIS
3. OTHER AUTOIMMUNE DISEASES
4. VASCULITIS WITH LOW BLOOD FLOW TO BRAIN
SEE DIAGNOSTIC FLOW SHEET
IMMUNE PARALYSIS – SUSCEPTIBILITY TO INFECTION:
1. LOW ANTIBODY RESPONSE
2. LOW NATURAL KILLER [NK] CELLS.

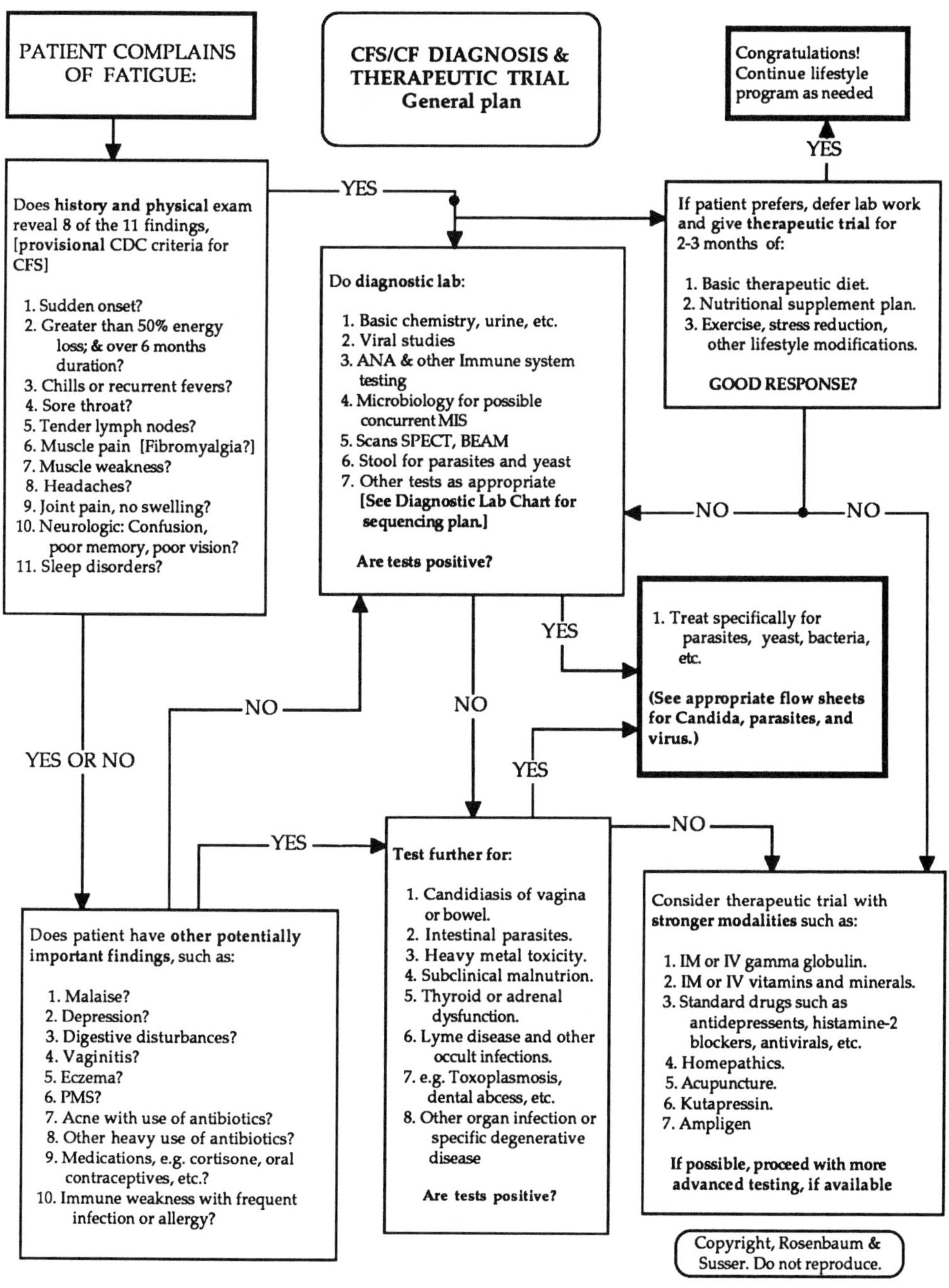
PATIENT COMPLAINS OF FATIGUE:
CFS/CF DIAGNOSIS & THERAPEUTIC TRIAL General plan
Congratulations! Continue lifestyle program as needed
YES
Does history and physical exam reveal 8 of the 11 findings, [provisional CDC criteria for CFS]
1. Sudden onset?
2. Greater than 50% energy loss; & over 6 months duration?
3. Chills or recurrent fevers?
4. Sore throat?
5. Tender lymph nodes?
6. Muscle pain [Fibromyalgia?]
7. Muscle weakness?
8. Headaches?
9. Joint pain, no swelling?
10. Neurologic: Confusion, poor memory, poor vision?
11. Sleep disorders?
YES
If patient prefers, defer lab work and give therapeutic trial for 2-3 months of:
1. Basic therapeutic diet.
2. Nutritional supplement plan.
3. Exercise, stress reduction, other lifestyle modifications.
GOOD RESPONSE?
Do diagnostic lab:
1. Basic chemistry, urine, etc.
2. Viral studies
3. ANA & other Immune system testing
4. Microbiology for possible concurrent MIS
5. Scans SPECT, BEAM
6. Stool for parasites and yeast
7. Other tests as appropriate [See Diagnostic Lab Chart for sequencing plan.]
Are tests positive?
NO
NO
YES
1. Treat specifically for parasites, yeast, bacteria, etc.
(See appropriate flow sheets for Candida, parasites, and virus.)
NO
NO
YES OR NO
YES
YES
NO
Test further for:
1. Candidiasis of vagina or bowel.
2. Intestinal parasites.
3. Heavy metal toxicity.
4. Subclinical malnutrion.
5. Thyroid or adrenal dysfunction.
6. Lyme disease and other occult infections.
7. e.g. Toxoplasmosis, dental abcess, etc.
8. Other organ infection or specific degenerative disease
Are tests positive?
Does patient have other potentially important findings, such as:
1. Malaise?
2. Depression?
3. Digestive disturbances?
4. Vaginitis?
5. Eczema?
6. PMS?
7. Acne with use of antibiotics?
8. Other heavy use of antibiotics?
9. Medications, e.g. cortisone, oral contraceptives, etc.?
10. Immune weakness with frequent infection or allergy?
Consider therapeutic trial with stronger modalities such as:
1. IM or IV gamma globulin.
2. IM or IV vitamins and minerals.
3. Standard drugs such as antidepressents, histamine-2 blockers, antivirals, etc.
4. Homepathics.
5. Acupuncture.
6. Kutapressin.
7. Ampligen
If possible, proceed with more advanced testing, if available
Copyright, Rosenbaum & Susser. Do not reproduce.

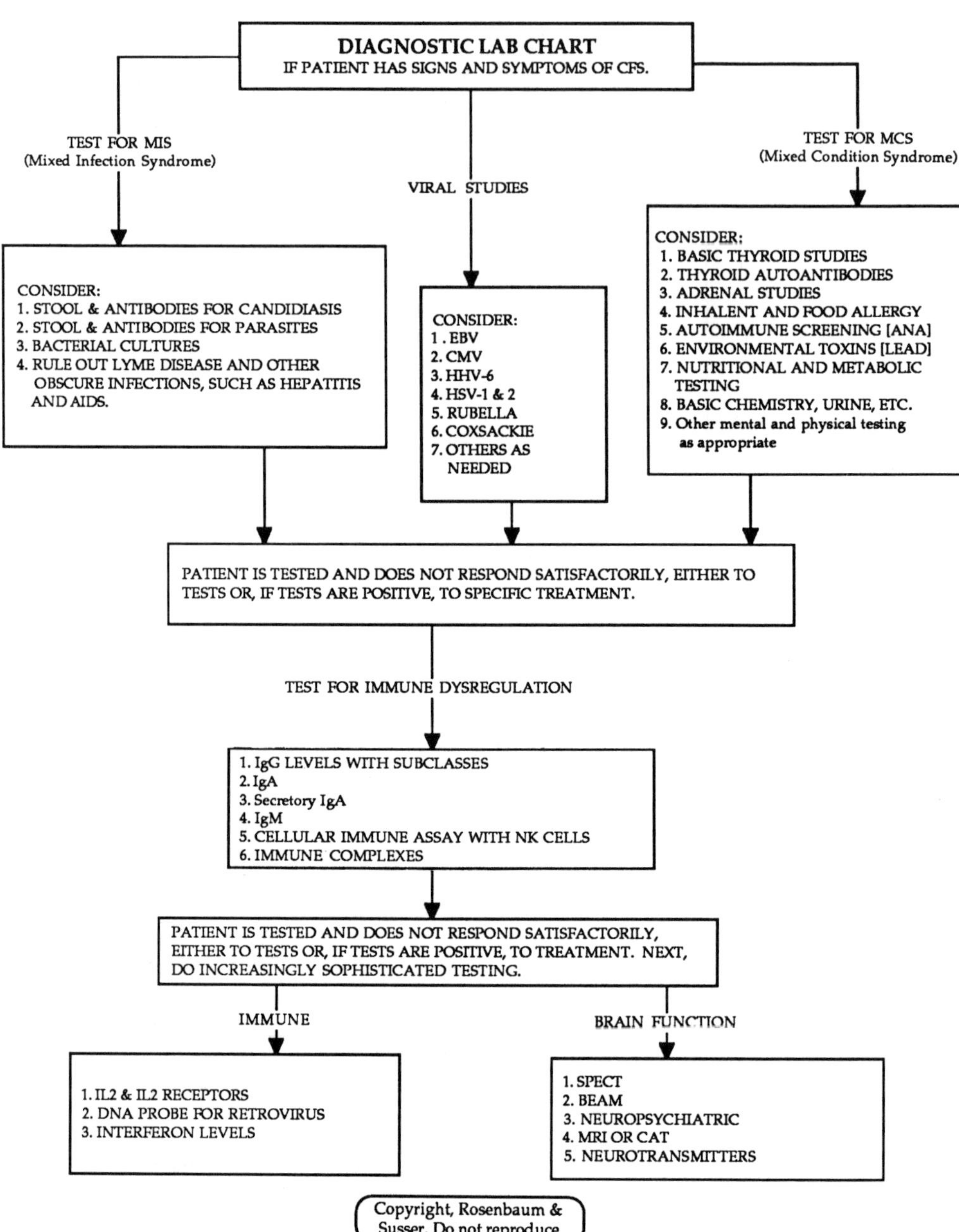
DIAGNOSTIC LAB CHART
IF PATIENT HAS SIGNS AND SYMPTOMS OF CFS.
TEST FOR MIS
(Mixed Infection Syndrome)
VIRAL STUDIES
TEST FOR MCS
(Mixed Condition Syndrome)
CONSIDER:
1. STOOL & ANTIBODIES FOR CANDIDIASIS
2. STOOL & ANTIBODIES FOR PARASITES
3. BACTERIAL CULTURES
4. RULE OUT LYME DISEASE AND OTHER OBSCURE INFECTIONS, SUCH AS HEPATITIS AND AIDS.
CONSIDER:
1. EBV
2. CMV
3. HHV-6
4. HSV-1 & 2
5. RUBELLA
6. COXSACKIE
7. OTHERS AS NEEDED
CONSIDER:
1. BASIC THYROID STUDIES
2. THYROID AUTOANTIBODIES
3. ADRENAL STUDIES
4. INHALENT AND FOOD ALLERGY
5. AUTOIMMUNE SCREENING [ANA]
6. ENVIRONMENTAL TOXINS [LEAD]
7. NUTRITIONAL AND METABOLIC TESTING
8. BASIC CHEMISTRY, URINE, ETC.
9. Other mental and physical testing as appropriate
PATIENT IS TESTED AND DOES NOT RESPOND SATISFACTORILY, EITHER TO TESTS OR, IF TESTS ARE POSITIVE, TO SPECIFIC TREATMENT.
TEST FOR IMMUNE DYSREGULATION
1. IgG LEVELS WITH SUBCLASSES
2. IgA
3. Secretory IgA
4. IgM
5. CELLULAR IMMUNE ASSAY WITH NK CELLS
6. IMMUNE COMPLEXES
PATIENT IS TESTED AND DOES NOT RESPOND SATISFACTORILY, EITHER TO TESTS OR, IF TESTS ARE POSITIVE, TO TREATMENT. NEXT, DO INCREASINGLY SOPHISTICATED TESTING.
IMMUNE
BRAIN FUNCTION
1. IL2 & IL2 RECEPTORS
2. DNA PROBE FOR RETROVIRUS
3. INTERFERON LEVELS
1. SPECT
2. BEAM
3. NEUROPSYCHIATRIC
4. MRI OR CAT
5. NEUROTRANSMITTERS

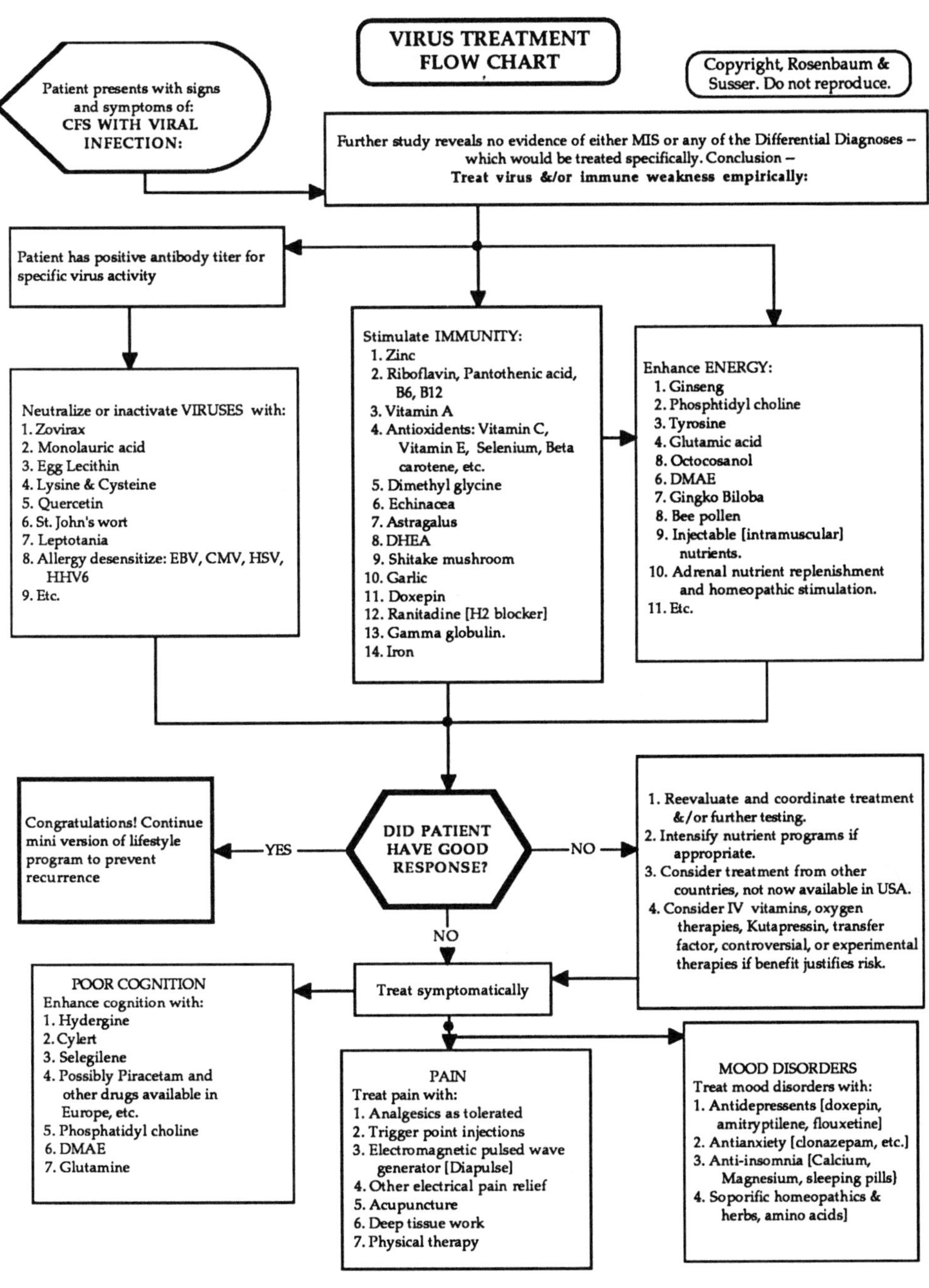
VIRUS TREATMENT FLOW CHART
Copyright, Rosenbaum & Susser. Do not reproduce.
Patient presents with signs and symptoms of: CFS WITH VIRAL INFECTION:
Further study reveals no evidence of either MIS or any of the Differential Diagnoses – which would be treated specifically. Conclusion – Treat virus &/or immune weakness empirically:
Patient has positive antibody titer for specific virus activity
Neutralize or inactivate VIRUSES with:
1. Zovirax
2. Monolauric acid
3. Egg Lecithin
4. Lysine & Cysteine
5. Quercetin
6. St. John's wort
7. Leptotania
8. Allergy desensitize: EBV, CMV, HSV, HHV6
9. Etc.
Stimulate IMMUNITY:
1. Zinc
2. Riboflavin, Pantothenic acid, B6, B12
3. Vitamin A
4. Antioxidents: Vitamin C, Vitamin E, Selenium, Beta carotene, etc.
5. Dimethyl glycine
6. Echinacea
7. Astragalus
8. DHEA
9. Shitake mushroom
10. Garlic
11. Doxepin
12. Ranitadine [H2 blocker]
13. Gamma globulin.
14. Iron
Enhance ENERGY:
1. Ginseng
2. Phosphtidyl choline
3. Tyrosine
4. Glutamic acid
8. Octocosanol
6. DMAE
7. Gingko Biloba
8. Bee pollen
9. Injectable [intramuscular] nutrients.
10. Adrenal nutrient replenishment and homeopathic stimulation.
11. Etc.
DID PATIENT HAVE GOOD RESPONSE?
YES
NO
Congratulations! Continue mini version of lifestyle program to prevent recurrence
1. Reevaluate and coordinate treatment &/or further testing.
2. Intensify nutrient programs if appropriate.
3. Consider treatment from other countries, not now available in USA.
4. Consider IV vitamins, oxygen therapies, Kutapressin, transfer factor, controversial, or experimental therapies if benefit justifies risk.
NO
Treat symptomatically
POOR COGNITION
Enhance cognition with:
1. Hydergine
2. Cylert
3. Selegilene
4. Possibly Piracetam and other drugs available in Europe, etc.
5. Phosphatidyl choline
6. DMAE
7. Glutamine
PAIN
Treat pain with:
1. Analgesics as tolerated
2. Trigger point injections
3. Electromagnetic pulsed wave generator [Diapulse]
4. Other electrical pain relief
5. Acupuncture
6. Deep tissue work
7. Physical therapy
MOOD DISORDERS
Treat mood disorders with:
1. Antidepressents [doxepin, amitryptilene, flouxetine]
2. Antianxiety [clonazepam, etc.]
3. Anti-insomnia [Calcium, Magnesium, sleeping pills]
4. Soporific homeopathics & herbs, amino acids]

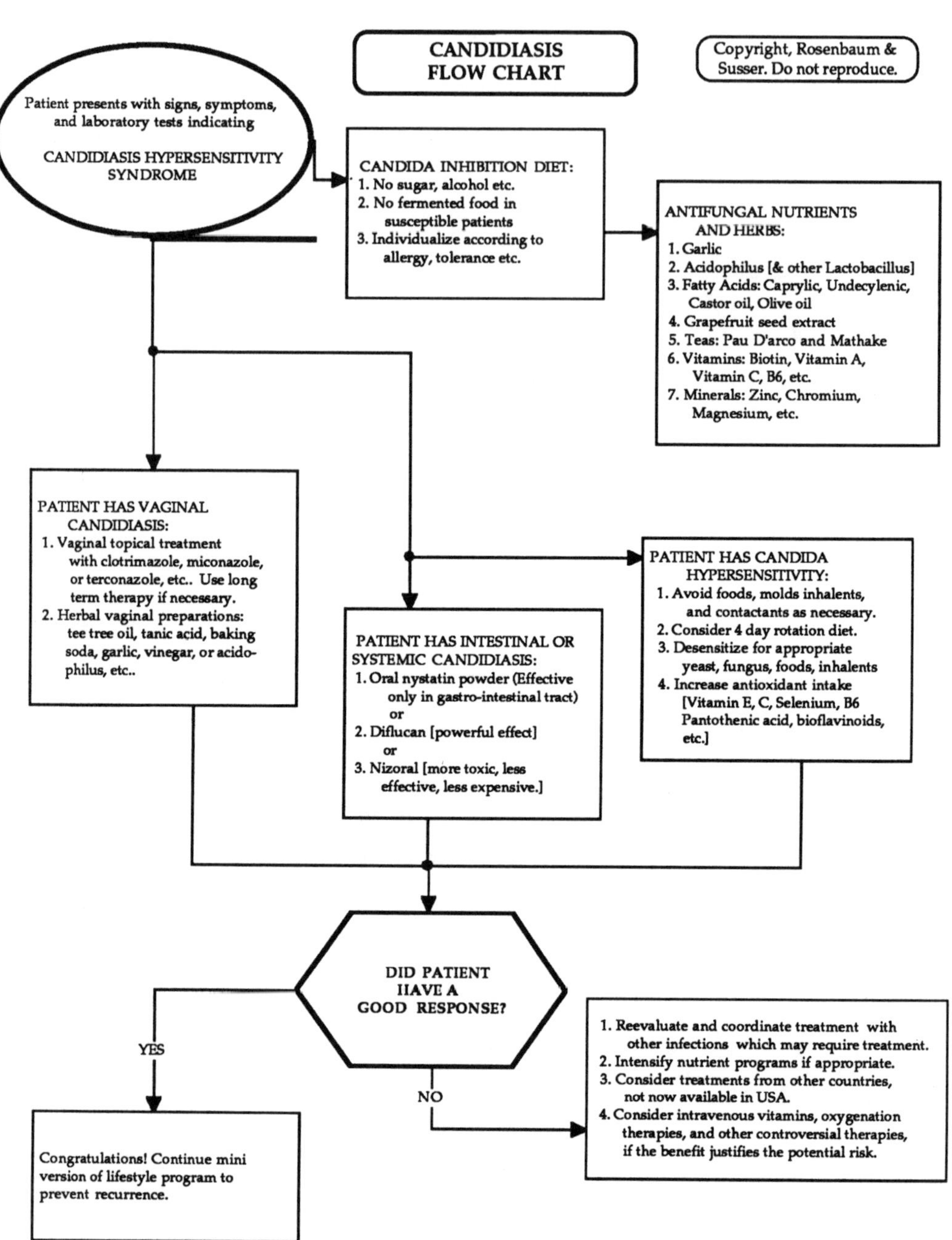
CANDIDIASIS
FLOW CHART
Copyright, Rosenbaum & Susser. Do not reproduce.
Patient presents with signs, symptoms, and laboratory tests indicating
CANDIDIASIS HYPERSENSITIVITY SYNDROME
CANDIDA INHIBITION DIET:
1. No sugar, alcohol etc.
2. No fermented food in susceptible patients
3. Individualize according to allergy, tolerance etc.
ANTIFUNGAL NUTRIENTS AND HERBS:
1. Garlic
2. Acidophilus [& other Lactobacillus]
3. Fatty Acids: Caprylic, Undecylenic, Castor oil, Olive oil
4. Grapefruit seed extract
5. Teas: Pau D'arco and Mathake
6. Vitamins: Biotin, Vitamin A, Vitamin C, B6, etc.
7. Minerals: Zinc, Chromium, Magnesium, etc.
PATIENT HAS VAGINAL CANDIDIASIS:
1. Vaginal topical treatment with clotrimazole, miconazole, or terconazole, etc.. Use long term therapy if necessary.
2. Herbal vaginal preparations: tee tree oil, tanic acid, baking soda, garlic, vinegar, or acidophilus, etc..
PATIENT HAS CANDIDA HYPERSENSITIVITY:
1. Avoid foods, molds inhalents, and contactants as necessary.
2. Consider 4 day rotation diet.
3. Desensitize for appropriate yeast, fungus, foods, inhalents
4. Increase antioxidant intake [Vitamin E, C, Selenium, B6 Pantothenic acid, bioflavinoids, etc.]
PATIENT HAS INTESTINAL OR SYSTEMIC CANDIDIASIS:
1. Oral nystatin powder (Effective only in gastro-intestinal tract)
or
2. Diflucan [powerful effect]
or
3. Nizoral [more toxic, less effective, less expensive.]
DID PATIENT HAVE A GOOD RESPONSE?
YES
NO
Congratulations! Continue mini version of lifestyle program to prevent recurrence.
1. Reevaluate and coordinate treatment with other infections which may require treatment.
2. Intensify nutrient programs if appropriate.
3. Consider treatments from other countries, not now available in USA.
4. Consider intravenous vitamins, oxygenation therapies, and other controversial therapies, if the benefit justifies the potential risk.

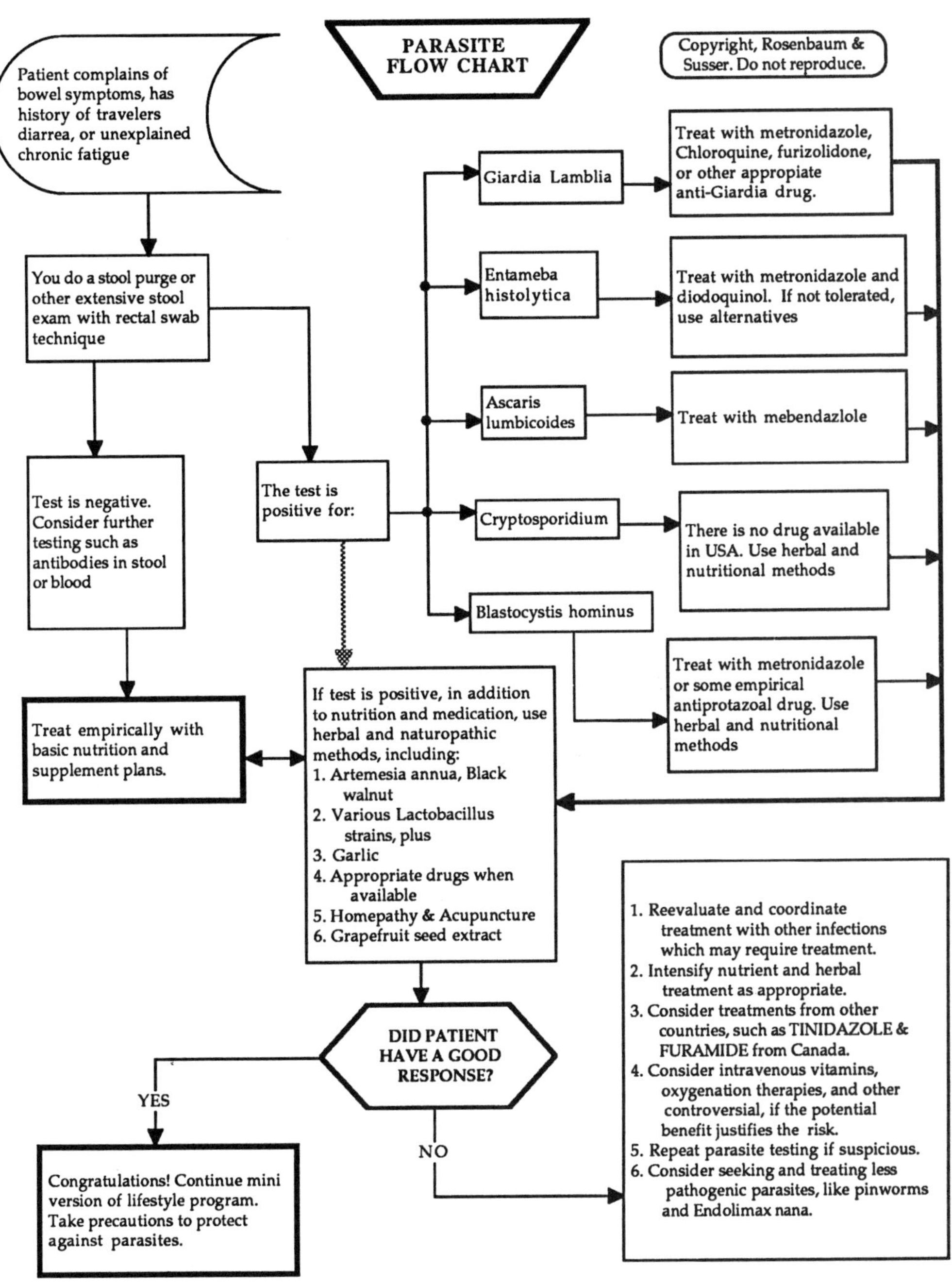
PARASITE FLOW CHART
Copyright, Rosenbaum & Susser. Do not reproduce.
Patient complains of bowel symptoms, has history of travelers diarrea, or unexplained chronic fatigue
You do a stool purge or other extensive stool exam with rectal swab technique
Test is negative. Consider further testing such as antibodies in stool or blood
The test is positive for:
Giardia Lamblia
Treat with metronidazole, Chloroquine, furizolidone, or other appropiate anti-Giardia drug.
Entameba histolytica
Treat with metronidazole and diodoquinol. If not tolerated, use alternatives
Ascaris lumbicoides
Treat with mebendazlole
Cryptosporidium
There is no drug available in USA. Use herbal and nutritional methods
Blastocystis hominus
Treat with metronidazole or some empirical antiprotazoal drug. Use herbal and nutritional methods
Treat empirically with basic nutrition and supplement plans.
If test is positive, in addition to nutrition and medication, use herbal and naturopathic methods, including:
1. Artemesia annua, Black walnut
2. Various Lactobacillus strains, plus
3. Garlic
4. Appropriate drugs when available
5. Homepathy & Acupuncture
6. Grapefruit seed extract
DID PATIENT HAVE A GOOD RESPONSE?
YES
NO
Congratulations! Continue mini version of lifestyle program. Take precautions to protect against parasites.
1. Reevaluate and coordinate treatment with other infections which may require treatment.
2. Intensify nutrient and herbal treatment as appropriate.
3. Consider treatments from other countries, such as TINIDAZOLE & FURAMIDE from Canada.
4. Consider intravenous vitamins, oxygenation therapies, and other controversial, if the potential benefit justifies the risk.
5. Repeat parasite testing if suspicious.
6. Consider seeking and treating less pathogenic parasites, like pinworms and Endolimax nana.

NEW FINDINGS ON CHRONIC FATIGUE SYNDROME

CFS CONFERENCE UPDATE, 1991

We were privileged to attend and address the CFS Conference covered in Los Angles in May of 1991. Among those present were medical luminaries in the fight against CFS: Dr. Jay Goldstein who sponsored and coordinated the conference, and Dr. Paul Cheney and Dr. Daniel Peterson who both confronted the Lake Tahoe Epidemic in 1984 that alerted the world to the CFS problem.

Summary of Conference Highlights

1. Too much RNAase

Brain cells and lymphocytes of CFS patients have enormous amounts of an enzyme called RNAase which destroys RNA genetic material. This enzyme increases modestly during ordinary viral infections as a non-specific protection against viruses, most of which contain RNA. It appears that RNAase production remains continually steep in CFS and has the potential to destroy brain and lymphocyte genetic material causing an immune dysregulation and a disruption of memory encoding. In addition, the process of overproducing RNAase consumes an excess of ATP, the "energy packets" of our cells, and has the potential to cause chronic fatigue. Should the RNAase theory be corroborated by extensive laboratory testing, it would provide a simple unified mechanism to explain the combination of unrelenting profound fatigue, impaired memory, and immune dysregulation found in CFS.

2. Low Blood Perfusion to the Brain

SPECT scans of blood flow to the brain were conducted at the USC School of Medicine in patients with CFS and depression. CFS patients demonstrated consistently poor perfusion of three specific focal areas of the brain: The left temporal, left frontal and right parietal regions. These regions control verbal capacity, memory processing, the entire limbic area which controls emotions, and most basic vegetative functions along with the higher mind or the capacity to think. The SPECT scans in depressed patients indicated a uniform reduction in blood flow throughout the brain. This pattern is markedly different than the pattern of blood flow observed in CFS and should help to dispel the skeptics who state that CFS is the same disease as depression. In fact, several psychologists at the meeting reported that neuro-psychological tests of CFS patients reveal a "distinct neurometric profile." Dr. Jay Goldstein expounded in great detail his theory that CFS is primarily a disease of "limbic encephalopathy." The limbic system of the brain is a major pathway which intercedes in human emotion, memory, and most vegetative functions including appetite, temperature control, sexual desire, and hormone regulation. The limbic system also sends nerves into the thymus and exerts control over immune functions. Since the cells of the immune system and of the brain emerge from the same embryonic cells, they may both be susceptible to the same "agent X" that he postulates is the initial trigger for CFS and dysregulates both the immune system and the limbic system. He feels that the adverse effects on the brain can cause most of the physical and mental aberrations observed in CFS.

3. A Cytokine Disease

There was much support for the contention that CFS is largely "a cytokine disease." It was reported that injections of the cytokines, interleukin-2, and alpha interferon into healthy human subjects can reproduce all the symptoms of general malaise that occur in CFS: fever, headache, muscle aches and pains, depression and impaired mental capacity.

4. Ampligen® - A new Biological Response Modifier

Ampligen (HEM Research, Inc., Rockville, MD) is a biological response modifier made up of double stranded RNA. It is an offshoot of a former substance called "poly I poly C" that exhibited promising benefits in the fight against cancer a decade ago; however, it was scrapped due to an unacceptably high incidence of toxic reactions. Ampligen is the same substance with one change. It has a mismatched nucleic acid at every thirteenth position which reduces its toxic potential while retaining its immune stimulating characteristics. Ampligen has been shown to stimulate the immune cell that is deficient and weak in CFS: the natural killer or NK cell. In addition, it has demonstrated an ability to reduce excessive RNAase levels. It sounds like a wonder drug for CFS.

The first report on its purported efficacy in CFS patients was made in October, 1991 by one of its co-inventors, Dr. William Carter of Hahnemann University School of Medicine in Philadelphia (who is also affiliated with HEM Pharmaceuticals), at a meeting of the American Society for Microbiology. Preliminary indications based on a multi-centered trial is that Ampligen may relieve some of the significant symptoms associated with CFS such as severe fatigue and memory loss. However, some experts have suggested caution until these findings are published and additional studies are completed *and* confirmed by independent scientists. We await the release of additional data on Ampligen with hopeful expectations. Besides its significant cost, which can exceed $1,000 for month, there is as yet no data on side effects or long term benefits. It may be possible, for example, that the drug must be continued indefinitely to benefit the patient. Once discontinued the CFS may revert. We await the release of additional data with considerable anticipation and hope our expectations for this promising agent will not be diminished by conflicting clinical outcomes.

The CFIDS Association, Inc. which claims to be the "largest active", membership association in the United States dedicated to CFIDS (CFS), publishes a magazine and provides resources and lists of health care professionals working with CFS.

Their address is: P.O. Box 220398, Charlotte, NC, 28222-0398. Their telephone number is: 1-800-442-3437 When calling this number you will get an extensive tape message touting the organization and information on its new 900 number offering updated information and research on CFS. The charge for using this 900 number in the USA is $2.00 the first minute and $1.00 each additional minute.

GLOSSARY

acidophilus Common term for the "friendly" bacteria *Lactobacillus acidophilus* which colonize the gastrointestinal tract, particularly the bowel, and the vagina. Necessary to maintain healthy bowel flora.

adaptogen A therapeutic substance, such as an herb or nutrient, which acts to normalize body functions.

allergen A substance that causes an allergic reaction, more properly called an antigen.

Alzheimer's disease Also called presenile dementia. A progressive brain disease that occurs in persons 35 to 70 years of age, marked by generalized atrophy of the brain. Some of its major symptoms include disorientation, memory impairment, difficulty in walking, and speech disorders.

ameba A single cell organism (protazoa) which infects the bowel. Any protozoan of the genus *Amoeba.*

antibody A protein produced by the immune system in response to any antigen (foreign proteins, microorganisms such as viruses or bacteria, etc.).

antigen Any substance which precipitates an immune reaction with an antibody. Bacteria, virus, pollen, dust, mold and incompletely digested food are common antigens. Their presence in the bloodstream causes specific antibodies to attach to them, creating an immune complex.

ARC Stands for AIDS-related-complex.

asymptomatic Without symptoms.

Atabrine® [chloroquine] An anti-parasitic drug.

autoimmune An immune response which attacks the host's own organs. Allergy against self.

B-cell Same as B-lymphotcyte.

B-lymphocyte White blood cells manufactured by the bone marrow which, when stimulated by an antigen, produce antibodies.

Burkitt's lymphoma A type of cancer found predominantly in Africa.

Blastocystis hominis A controversial single cell organism which resides in the gut and may be either a parasite or a yeast.

bowel flora The microbes that populate the bowel.

candida Same as *Candida albicans.*

Candida albicans (C. *albicans*) A genus of yeastlike fungi. Yeast organism which can cause such infections as thrush (mouth), vaginitis, and systemic infections.

candidiasis Infection with the microrganisms of the genus *Candida.*

candida-hypersensitivity syndrome The allergic symptom complex which may accompany candida infection.

carcinogen A substance which causes cancer.

carcinogenesis The origin, development or production of cancer.

cellular immune system Immune system reactions involving macrophages and T-cells.
cell-mediated immunity Same as cellular immune system.
CF Chronic fatigue.
CFIDS Chronic fatigue immune difficiency syndrome.
CFS Chronic fatigue syndrome.
chelation therapy The use of metal binding agents to remove heavy metals and such trace elements as calcium from the body.
CMV Cytomegalovirus.
complement A system of protein molecules which circulate in the blood and which are activated by emergencies such as the presence of immune complexes. A series of reactions follow which bring a number of other cell types into the general immune response, causing inflammation and increased local concentration of T cells and B cells. Complement proteins are also able to kill foreign cells by piercing the cell membrane.
cystitis Inflamation of the urinary bladder.
cytomegalovirus A herpes family virus sometimes associated with CFS. It has a special affinity for the salvary glands. Sometimes also called salivary gland virus and herpesvirus 5.

dimorphic Having two distinct forms.
dehydroascorbic acid The oxidized (destroyed) form of ascorbic acid (vitamin C).
deoxyribonucleic acid The molecular basis of heredity. The genetic material which makes up the double helix in the nucleus of the cell.
DNA Deoxyribonucleic acid.
dysbiosis Imbalance of flora wherever they may reside.

EBV A herpes family virus sometimes associated with CFS.
E. coli A non-pathogenic form of the genus amebae found in the intestinal tract of man. Also called *Amoeba coli.*
endogenous From within. Generally in medicine refers to something found in the body.
Entameba histolytica A single cell organism (protazoa) which infects the bowel. Can cause amebic dysentery and amebic abscess of the liver. It can invade the the bowel mucosa causing ulceration and may be carried to other organs by the blood.
environmental illness Hypersensitivity to environmental chemicals, gases, etc.
epidemiology The study of public health; the origin and important characteristics of disease in populations.
epithelium The layer of cells lining the surface of all passages within the body, especially those which are open to the outside, such as the nasal and oral cavity, the throat, respiratory tract, gastrointestinal tract, vagina and cervix.
Epstein Barr virus Named after Alois Epstein, M.D A herpes-like virus that causes an infection similar to mononucleosis.
ESR [sed rate] Blood test indicating non-specific inflammation.
exogenous External source. Something that comes from outside the body.

Flagyl® [metronidazole] Drug used to kill parasites and certain bacteria.
free radical An unstable molecular fragment with an unpaired (missing) electron that can potentially cause damage to bodily cells.
Furoxone® [furizolidone] Drug used to kill parasites and certain bacteria.

gamma globulin The antibody containing fraction of the blood.
Giardia lamblia A single cell organism (protozoa) which infects the bowel.
glycohemoglobin Blood test which screens for diabetes and low blood sugar.

Hashimoto's disease Autoimmune thyroid and lymph inflammation.
Herpesvirus A family of hibernating viruses, widespread in humans, which may be suppressed by the immune system but rarely eradicated.
HIV Human immunodeficiency virus. The pathogenic agent thought to be the primary cause of ARC and AIDS. Formerally known as HTLV-III.
HSV Herpes simplex virus.
humoral immune system Immune system reactions involving B-cells and the antibodies they produce.
hypersensitivity Excess sensitivity to foreign proteins and agents.

Ig immunoglobulin Synonym for antibody.
IM Infectious mononucleosis.
infectious mononucleosis A debilitating infection which involves the throat, liver, much of lymphatic tissues of the body. Sometimes called the "kissing disease."
immune complex disease A hypersensitivity reaction marked by deposition of antigen-antibody complement complexes within tissues, especially in the vascular endothelium.
immune system The state that allows the body to recognize agents as foreign to itself and to proceed to neutralize, eliminate or metabolize them with or without injury to surrounding tissue.
interferon A class of lymphokines, specialized proteins, produced by the immune system which warn uninfected cells of viral invasion, stimulate the activity of T-cells and NK cells, and help prevent viruses from penetrating healthy cells. Sometimes abbreviated INF.
interleukin usually specified by number, IL-1 through 6. Small proteins made by white blood cells to stimulate other blood cells.
in vitro Occuring under external laboratory conditions, such as in a test tube.
in vivo Occuring within a living organism, usually the human body.
invasive Penetrating the superficial layers of exposure.
IV Intravenous.

Lactobacillus acidophilus The "friendly" bacteria which colonize the bowel and the vagina.
lipid The chemical/medical name for fats and oils.
lumen The hollow center of an organ such as the bowel or a blood vessel.
lupus One of several autoimmune disorders, the most common of which is called systemic lupus erythematosis. Autoimmune disease in which the body attacks its own connective tissue.

lymphocyte An immune cell, also known as white blood cells. There are two major types of lymphocytes. B-lymphocytes and T-lymphocytes (T-cells).
lymphokine A macrophage; literally big [macro] eater [phage].
lysis The piercing or bursting of a cell.

microbe Any microscopic organism, including viruses, bacteria, parasites and yeast.
microsome An organelle within the cell.
MIS Mixed Infection Syndrome.
mixed infection syndrome Debilitating disease, characterized by more than one organism simultaneously infecting the body.
MRI Magnetic resonance imaging. A magnetic computerized diagnostic scan of a selected region of the body.
MS Multiple Sclerosis.
mutagen A substance which causes cells to mutate, often leading to increased risk of cancer.

nasopharyngeal Referring to the area of the throat and nasal passages.
natural killer cells Also abbreviated as NK cells. A subset of T-cells which are capable of destroying foreign substances without first becoming activated. NK cells, in addition, do not need antibody "tags" to recognize invaders. NK cell activity is enhanced by interferon and IL-2.
NK cells Natural killer cells.
NPC Nasopharyngeal carcinoma.
nasopharyngeal carcinoma A type of cancer beginning in the nasopharynx and commonly associated with the EBV.

oxidative therapies The therepeutic use of reactive forms of oxygen such as hydrogen peroxide and ozone, as well as high concentration and high pressure oxygen.

parasites Organisms which live off other organisms. Also, certain microbes which are not bacteria, fungus, or virus that generally cause tropical/sub-tropical diseases.
passive immunity Protection derived from exogenous and therefore temporary sources, such as gamma globulin.
pathogen A disease-producing organism.
PEM Protein energy malnutrition.
peptide A link between amino acids.
phagocytosis The engulfing of pathogens by cells such as macrophages or neutrophils.
primary infection Infection resulting from the first exposure to a pathogen. In the case of Epstein-Barr virus, primary infection usually takes place in childhood, and produces no noticeable symptoms.
protozoa A single cell parasitic organism.

serology The study of blood serum, especially relating to immunity and the presence of antibodies.

seronegative Serum which does not contain antibodies to a specific antigen, indicating that infection by that antigen has not taken place, or that the body failed to develop antibodies.
seropositive Serum which contains antibodies to a specific antigen, indicating that infection by that antigen has taken place. Also the synovial fluid, a mucin-containing liquid which lubricates joints or the surface of some tendons.
SLE Systemic lupus erythematosis. See Lupus.
stress The non-specific response of the body to any demand put upon it.
synovium The tissue which lines and encompasses the joints.
systemic lupus erythematosis See Lupus.

thymus gland The master control of the immune system, residing under the breast bone.
transfer factor Immunologic "soup" produced from special treatment of white blood cells. Used to treat CFS and other immune weaknesses.

VCA Viral capsid antigen. A specific immune marker antibody.
virion A single virus organism.

Yodoxin® [iodoquinol] Drug used to kill parasites.

INDEX